The Mind's Whisper: Recognizing Early Signs of Cognitive Decline

Ravi

Table of Contents

Introduction

As the global population ages and pathological cognitive decline in late-life becomes a more predominant clinical concern (Canadian Institutes of Health Research, 2013), dementia research has been increasingly dedicated to identifying the earliest potential signs of incipient neurodegeneration. Given the intractability of dementia once established, the hope remains that identification of conversion risk at an early juncture may increase the effectiveness of cognitive interventions and preventative efforts. In service to this goal, the developmental window of interest has increasingly shifted backward: a primary focus on fully-realized Alzheimer's disease (AD) gave way to interest in early AD, then mild cognitive impairment (MCI), and even early MCI (Edmonds et al., 2019; Jessen et al., 2014). Most recently, subjective cognitive decline (SCD) has been identified as the potential earliest indicator of cognitive risk (Imtiaz, Tolppanen, Kivipelto, & Soininen, 2014; Smart et al., 2017).

Unlike MCI, which is defined by objective cognitive declines despite the maintenance of functional independence (Jessen et al., 2014), SCD constitutes self-reported cognitive decline in spite of objective cognitive performance within the expected range (Jessen et al., 2020). At its core, SCD represents a fundamental schism between individuals' experience of their own abilities and the outcomes of objective evaluation measures. Given the regularity of cognitive complaints in older adulthood (Cooper et al., 2011; Jonker, Geerlings, & Schmand, 2000), objective measures have historically been considered the more accurate and clinically significant source of data; however, the results of more recent work have called this clinical wisdom into question. Specifically, there is evidence to suggest that, for some, SCD may indeed augur objective cognitive declines and conversion to dementia (Reisberg, Shulman, Torossian, Leng, & Zhu, 2010). Building on this, the endorsement of SCD has been linked with AD-consistent pathophysiological markers (e.g., Cherbuin, Sargent-Cox, Easteal, Sachdev, & Anstey, 2015; Stewart et al., 2011) and genetic risk factors (e.g., Ali, Smart, & Gawryluk, 2018). In light of these findings and the proposed chronology from SCD to frank dementia (Jessen, Amariglio, et al., 2014), SCD has been considered as a potentially useful index of susceptibility to dementia conversion or even the earliest manifestation of developing neuropathological processes (Buckley et al., 2016; Lista et al., 2015). Despite its clinical potential, however, the widescale adoption of SCD as a consistent and meaningful index for dementia risk has been undermined by several fundamental challenges.

Conceptual Challenges to Adoption of SCD as a Standalone Dementia Risk Index

Aetiological heterogeneity. Chief among these challenges is the multi-determined nature of SCD. In recent years, it has become clear that prodromal conditions like MCI and, potentially SCD, lack diagnostic specificity and connote more general risk for developing objective cognitive decline and indeterminate pathology (Tuokko & Smart, 2018). Despite its association with pathological processes, (Ali et al., 2018), SCD endorsement is also highly correlated with psychological factors, such as trait neuroticism, anxiety, and depression (Comijs, Deeg, Dik, Twisk, & Jonker, 2002; Derouesné, Lacomblez, Thibault, & LePoncin, 1999; Dux et al., 2008; Slavin et al., 2010). Multi-determined themselves, these psychological factors may be exacerbated by yet other influences (e.g., Allaz & Cedraschi, 2015; Gibson, 2015; Goesling, Clauw, & Hassett, 2013). When combined with the fact that normatively aging older adults also endorse cognitive changes, disentangling SCD that is potentially prodromal from SCD due to other factors becomes a complicated matter indeed (Tuokko & Smart, 2018).

Definition and terminology. Yet another challenge is the historically wide range of SCD conceptualizations. This heterogeneity is perhaps reflected best by terminology used for SCD and equivalent conditions across the literature (Ali et al., 2018; Rabin et al., 2015). Terms as diverse as "cognitive complaints", "subjective cognitive concerns", "memory complaints", "subjective memory concerns", "subjective memory impairment", "subjective cognitive impairment", and the more recent "subjective cognitive decline" have all been used to describe relatively equivalent clinical constructs – that is, self-perceived change in cognitive ability belied by intact performance on objective tests. As part and parcel of this conceptual chaos, clinicians and researchers alike have struggled to identify which symptoms and aspects of SCD are clinically significant. Earlier definitions of SCD focused exclusively on perceived memory decline owing to the AD-specific lens employed at the time. Although more recent SCD conceptualizations acknowledge the potential import of other cognitive domains, many research groups continue to persist with memory-specific definitions. The lack of standardization in SCD research makes it difficult to synthesize our knowledge and build consensus around "true" SCD-related risk for dementia.

Related, a subtle but significant terminological difference between "complaints" and "concerns" has further muddied the diagnostic waters. Cognitive complaints and cognitive concerns have traditionally been viewed as equivalent and interchangeable; however, there is evidence to suggest that these two symptoms may relate to fundamentally unique aspects of aging. While the majority of older adults endorse some degree of cognitive complaints (Jonker et al., 2000), a much smaller proportion report concern or worry that their perceived cognitive changes are beyond what would be expected for someone their age, or that their experiences may be suggestive of a pathological process. Supporting this distinction, the large-scale AgeCoDe study found that it was the presence of concern and not merely the endorsement of complaints that was associated with the greatest risk of dementia conversion (Jessen et al., 2010; Wolfsgruber et al., 2016).

Categorical vs. continuous conceptualizations. Yet another aspect of SCD that has proven contentious is whether it ought to be viewed – and consequently, measured – as a continuous or categorical variable. Historically, cognitive complaints (broadly defined) were characterized according to their number, frequency, or intensity. In this way, researchers aimed to determine a clinically-relevant diagnostic threshold for high-risk vs. age-normative experiences of cognitive change. While intuitively sound, this approach has been called into question in light of recent evidence that the mere presence of SCD is sufficient to impart cognitive risk (Jessen et al., 2014). As a result, Alzheimer's Disease Centers across North America have begun to identify SCD using a single categorical item: "Does the subject report a decline in memory relative to previously attained abilities?" (Kielb, Rogalski, Weintraub, & Rademaker, 2017). Nevertheless, classification methods remain diverse (Rabin et al., 2015), with SCD variously conceptualized as a singular construct (e.g., Jessen et al., 2014) or a continuous variable (e.g., Verlinden et al., 2017) depending on study aims, research setting (e.g., memory clinic), and researcher preference.

Practical Challenges to Determining SCD-Related Risk for Dementia

Standardized cognitive/neuropsychological assessment. The lack of conceptual consensus around SCD has made it challenging to build a unified body of knowledge regarding when and how SCD confers risk. As an extension of these underlying issues, determining how best to assess SCD-related vulnerability has also proven contentious. By definition, those with SCD achieve scores within normal limits on standardized tests (Jessen et al., 2014); however, quantitatively-minded researchers have continued to probe the performance profiles of those with SCD for any recognizable patterns of cognitive strength and weakness that might prove predictive of dementia. Laudable though these efforts may be, they have met with limited success thus far. Notably, the challenge has not been the lack of significant outcomes, but the lack of cohesive and consistent findings. For instance, SCD endorsers have been found to perform more poorly than those without SCD on cognitive screening measures (Stewart et al., 2001), as well as clinical tests of simple attention (Fortea et al., 2011), memory (Jessen et al., 2007), and executive functioning (Fonseca et al., 2015); however, these results remain inconsistently replicated due to marked heterogeneity in sample characteristics, assessment approaches/tools, and research paradigms (Ali et al., 2018). Yet another likely contributor may simply be the psychometric properties of standardized clinical-neuropsychological measures. By design, such tests excel at identifying cognitive performance within the frankly impaired range but at the expense of being relatively *insensitive* to incremental differences within normal-range performance (e.g., SCD).

Self-report measures. Due to the aforementioned shortcomings of objective standardized cognitive-neuropsychological assessment, efforts to characterize SCD have primarily relied upon self-report measures. Unfortunately, self-report measures suffer from many of the same issues of insensitivity, lack of specificity, and general lack of clinical consensus (Rabin et al., 2015) that plague other quantitative tests. Particularly relevant to SCD and the SCD *Plus* criteria (Jessen et al., 2014), few self-report measures differentiate between assessing the occurrence of perceived cognitive declines, the perceived normativity of cognitive declines experienced, and the degree of concern resulting from perceived cognitive changes. Consequently, it has proven difficult to determine exactly what "SCD" means across various studies. Related, there is little consensus regarding which measures are most relevant for identifying dementia-predicting SCD, or even what form such a tool should take. Extremely diverse methods have been implemented across studies, which include classifying anyone presenting to clinic with concerns as having SCD (e.g., Sierra-Rio et al., 2016); asking single questions about perceived declines in memory (Kielb et al., 2017) or cognitive changes more generally (e.g., Hall et al., 2015); asking single questions about concern due to perceived cognitive changes (e.g., Dhilla Albers et al., 2016); or administering various self-report measures (e.g., Mattsson et al., 2015; Risacher et al., 2015). Without the development of reliable SCD-specific items/measures and standardized diagnostic methods, SCD will continue to be an underutilized source of potentially crucial clinical information. As it stands currently, self-report measures in isolation may be unsuitable for disentangling normative age-related experiences of cognitive change from potentially pathological SCD (Rabin et al., 2015).

Qualitative enquiry. Very few studies of the first-person experience of individuals with SCD have been undertaken. Clinical researchers commonly administer self-report measures designed for cognitively impaired populations to those with SCD; however, lacking any real understanding of the subjective experience of SCD, it remains unclear whether these measures truly represent the issues of most personal salience or diagnostic significance for those with SCD. These sentiments are far from novel and have been echoed by prominent voices in SCD research (Buckley, Saling, Frommann, Wolfsgruber, & Wagner, 2015; Rabin et al., 2015). Potentially more powerful yet, qualitative approaches represent a direct corollary to actual clinical interactions. As frontline clinicians are likely to be presented with subjective accounts of cognitive change and concern, there would be exceptional benefit in determining key qualitative indicators of cognitive risk. At the least, such information would allow clinicians to better determine the need for advanced evaluation and intervention. Unfortunately, the few qualitative studies on SCD available have demonstrated that qualitative methods alone may be insufficient to provide the clear guidance required for diagnosis and intervention planning. The qualitative approaches taken to date (i.e., phenomenology) are idiosyncratic in nature and garner outcomes that are too broad and ambiguous to build reliable clinical practice upon (Creswell & Poth, 2017). However, this is not to say that qualitative methods as a whole are ill-equipped for such an undertaking. For instance, grounded theory approaches employ a more structured approach to data collection and interpretation that correspond well with more traditional quantitative paradigms. Unfortunately, such an approach have yet to be applied to SCD.

Rationale for a mixed-methods approach. Overall, SCD shows promise as one of the earliest prodromes of AD and other late-life cognitive pathology. However, its study and, until recently, definition, has been lacking in cohesiveness. This in turn has undermined efforts to capitalize on the clinical potential that SCD represents. Taken together, cognitive-neuropsychological assessment, self-report, and qualitative interviewing each appear to provide unique and valuable information regarding the effects and experiences of SCD; however, in isolation, each of these methods have also proven insufficient for characterizing SCD as a whole or distinguishing high-risk SCD in particular. With this in mind, a mixed-methods approach combining these various sources of information may be timely. The combined use of these methods may serve to bridge traditionally isolated areas of SCD research and make clearer how known risk factors interact. In other words, the use of a mixed-methods approach may make it possible to create an integrated multi-modal risk profile that is useful for clinicians and researchers alike.

Potential Risk Factors and Variables of Interest

Subjective cognitive decline criteria: SCD *Plus*. The SCD-Initiative Working Group has developed research criteria as an attempt to standardize SCD classification and identify persons with SCD at highest risk of developing into AD or other objective cognitive impairment (SCD *Plus*; Jessen et al., 2014). This criteria establishes a more inclusive definition of SCD that accommodates self-perceived decline across a number of cognitive domains, with special relevance of memory complaints to Alzheimer's pathology (Jessen et al., 2014; Molinuevo et al., 2017). According to the SCD *Plus* criteria, factors associated with the greatest likelihood of decline include: 1) subjective memory decline vs. decline in other cognitive domains; 2) SCD onset within the last 5 years; 3) SCD onset at age 60 or older; 4) concerns regarding cognitive decline; 5) feeling that one's cognitive abilities are worse than others the same age; 6) confirmation of decline by an informant; 7) presence of at least one APOE ε4 allele; and 8) biomarker evidence for AD. Currently, the SCD *Plus* framework provides the most nuanced and clinically-relevant classification of SCD available; however, its criteria remain relatively broad and do little to clarify critical items, relative weight of specific criteria, or diagnostic cut-offs/thresholds. Further, the

SCD *Plus* criteria may not represent the reality of clinical presentation or practice, where APOE ε4 genotype, family reports, and other information may remain absent, undisclosed, or difficult to access. Thus, although the SCD *Plus* framework provides the most integrated, comprehensive, and data-driven means of SCD risk classification to date, it remains insufficient for guiding clinical decision making. The development of novel, accessible, and easy-to-administer screening criteria that extend the SCD *Plus* framework into the clinical space may be an appropriate next step. In step with this goal and the SCD-Initiative Working Group's recommendations, the SCD *Plus* criteria served as the basis for SCD classification in each of the following studies (Chapters 3 and 4).

Objective cognitive decline criteria: Subtle cognitive decline. Unlike longitudinal studies that can track the development of frank impairment over time, single-point studies examining dementia potentiality in unimpaired samples (e.g., SCD) require concrete performance markers to define objective risk at the pre-clinical stage. Determining a suitable objective measure of cognitive decline in SCD samples is challenging due to the stipulation that individuals with SCD must perform within normal limits upon objective cognitive testing by definition. Further complicating matters, standardized tests tend to be insensitive to nuanced performance differences when scores fall within the normal range. Combined, the need to determine objective markers of decline and the difficulty defining and obtaining this data presents a theoretical and practical impasse; however, recent work applying the construct of "subtle cognitive decline" (subtle CD) may circumvent some of the issues.

The 2011 National Institute on Aging and the Alzheimer's Association (NIA-AA) research criteria for preclinical AD (Sperling et al., 2011) outlines three distinct AD risk factors, initially assumed to develop in a chronologically linear fashion: cerebral amyloid accumulation, advancing to neurodegeneration, and finally culminating in subtle CD as the last step before the onset of frank AD. However, no clear definition for subtle CD was provided in these guidelines. The construct of subtle CD added little to the clinical literature as a purely qualitative descriptor and, worse, was not amenable to examination due to its ambiguous nature. To remedy this, Edmonds and colleagues (Edmonds, Delano-Wood, Galasko, Salmon, & Bondi, 2015) provided an operational definition for use in their study.

Edmonds et al. (2015) administered a brief battery of six tests divided equally across three cognitive domains (i.e., memory, language, attention/executive function). For the purposes of their study, they defined individuals as demonstrating subtle CD when a single score in two of three cognitive domains fell >1 SD below the age-normed mean. They defined those with more than one low score within a given domain or with a single low score in each of the three domains to have probable MCI instead. Upon follow-up, they found subtle CD to occur relatively frequently in their sample of healthy older adults and, when paired with any other risk factor, to significantly increase the risk of eventually developing objective cognitive impairment. Though, perhaps not a sure risk indicator alone, subtle CD appeared to confer multiplicative risk for dementia when combined with amyloid deposition or neurodegeneration.

Based on these outcomes, subtle CD appears to be a good candidate for an objective risk indicator in the pre-clinical phases of possible neurodegeneration. Nevertheless, the criteria as outlined by Edmonds et al. (2015) does seem incompatible with more comprehensive test batteries that include more tests, more outcomes per test, and assess more cognitive domains. Thus, for the following studies (Chapters 3 and 4), we applied an amended version of Edmonds and colleagues' criteria for subtle CD. Given the regularity with which healthy older adults achieve lower than expected scores (Binder, Iverson, & Brooks, 2009) and the inflated potential of family-wise error in a larger test battery, we retained Edmonds et al.'s criteria for subtle CD but substituted their frequency-based criteria for probable MCI. Instead, we applied a percentage-based exclusionary criterion such that individuals were considered to have probable MCI rather than subtle CD only when >50% of scores within a given cognitive domain fall >1 standard deviation below the age-normative mean. We believe this amendment stays true to the intent of Edmonds et al.'s definition while allowing for its application to a more comprehensive battery. Like Edmonds et al.'s criteria, our operationalization of subtle CD was based on standardized cognitive-neuropsychological test performance alone. Although the NIA-AA criteria assumes that subtle CD is a precursor for objective decline, our cross-sectional study was not designed to test this. Further, due to the novelty of our operationalization, it is remains unclear whether the relationship between subtle CD and objective decline would be substantiated in our studies even if they were conducted longitudinally. As such, subtle CD in the following studies should be cautiously interpreted as a potential risk factor for objective decline rather than an established prodromal condition.

Genetic risk biomarker: APOE ε4 genotype. The clinical significance and reliability of our multi-method, convergent approach would be further bolstered by the inclusion of known genetic risk markers as these provide objective data relatively free from statistical error, psychometric shortcomings, or psychological contributions (e.g., anxiety). A prime candidate for this risk marker may be the ε4 variant of the APOE gene. Though many of these biomarkers (e.g., PiB-PET) are not easily accessible to clinicians outside major research centres, APOE ε4 genotype is easily obtained through low-cost non-invasive methods, and has shown promise in differentiating those with AD-predicting SCD from those with SCD associated with other etiologies (Krell-Roesch et al., 2015). APOE ε4 has been consistently identified as a risk factor for conversion to AD and vascular dementia (Allan & Ebmeier, 2011; Chen et al., 2016; Jiang et al., 2016; Liu et al., 2016; Mata et al., 2014; Pink et al., 2015; Prestia et al., 2015). APOE ε4 carriers have been estimated to have approximately three times greater risk of developing AD, while double allele carriers are estimated to be approximately 15 times more likely than the general population to develop AD (Farrer et al., 1997). With respect to SCD, a recent review found that APOE ε4 does not impact the development of SCD (broadly defined), but that SCD and APOE ε4 confer independent and interacting risk for conversion to an objectively impaired state (Ali et al., 2018). Further, APOE ε4-positive individuals with SCD were more likely to demonstrate cortical atrophy and amyloid deposition compared to healthy controls and APOE ε4-negative individuals (Ali et al., 2018). Given the relationship between SCD, APOE ε4, and AD-consistent pathology, APOE ε4 genotype may provide crucial insight into risk for cognitive decline among those with SCD and may contextualize otherwise ambiguous evidence provided through other approaches. It is for exactly this reason that both the SCD *Plus* guidelines for high-risk SCD (Jessen et al., 2014) and NIA preclinical AD criteria (Jack et al., 2018) encourage the collection of biomarker data to supplement neuropsychological test scores and self-reports.

book Overview and Objectives

Despite our compiled knowledge of risk-predicting complaints (e.g., Amariglio, Townsend, Grodstein, Sperling, & Rentz, 2011), underlying neuropathological symptoms (e.g., Striepens et al., 2010), and idiosyncratic cognitive test performance (Edmonds et al., 2015; Nikolai et al., 2018) in persons with SCD, none of this has coalesced into a "gold standard" measure or assessment method like those used to diagnose other conditions (e.g., MCI). In the absence of clear assessment direction, frontline clinicians may be exceptionally likely to overlook pertinent and early clinical signs. Accordingly, a mixed-methods approach leveraging convergent quantitative and qualitative risk indicators may be warranted to identify the specific characteristics of currently health older adults who may be at increased risk of eventual conversion to dementia.

Chapter 1. This chapter is a reproduction of a previously published article authored by the Principal Investigator and several Supervisory Committee members prior to the undertaking of the current book (Ali et al., 2018). This article presents a systematic review of the available literature regarding the relationship between APOE ε4 genotype and SCD. It is included in order to provide a comprehensive rationale for our inclusion of APOE ε4 genetic testing in the current studies and to contextualize the concluding discussion.

Chapter 2. This chapter provides a detailed overview of the methods and materials used for each of the studies performed for this book.

Chapter 3. The aim in this study was to clarify the relationship(s) between SCD, APOE ε4 genotype, specific psychosocial factors, and potential prodromal pathological cognitive decline (i.e., subtle CD). Of particular interest was whether SCD endorsement and subtle CD are influenced by the same factors and, by extension, to determine whether and how these two variables relate to one another. Given the non-specific aetiology of SCD discussed above, our first objective was to 1) isolate the specific psychosocial, cognitive, and genetic factors that contribute most to SCD endorsement. Next, we aimed to 2) clarify whether and to what extent SCD endorsement and APOE ε4 genotype relate to objective cognitive performance (i.e, subtle CD). Binary logistic regressions with stepwise entry were used for each of our analyses.

Chapter 4. The aim of this investigation was to determine which, if any, complaints, concerns, and/or experiences may be unique to high-risk older adults – that is, those who endorse SCD and/or who demonstrate subtle CD. Specifically, the primary objectives of this study was to 1) to determine which, if any, specific first-hand cognitive aging experiences were associated with SCD and subtle CD. As an auxiliary outcome, we expected to generate a list of potential screening items that might be easily probed during routine clinical interactions. Qualitative interviews were conducted with all participants and the data transcribed. Transcribed data was then qualitatively

coded, assigned a numeric label, and analyze via statistical means. APOE ε4 genotype was not

included as a variable of interest in this study due to the low *n* of APOE ε4-positive individuals in

our sample.

References

Ali, J. I., Smart, C. M., & Gawryluk, J. R. (2018). Subjective cognitive decline and APOE E4: A systematic review. *Journal of Alzheimer's Disease, 65*(1), 303–320.

Allan, C. L., & Ebmeier, K. P. (2011). The influence of ApoE4 on clinical progression of dementia: a meta-analysis. *International Journal of Geriatric Psychiatry, 26*(5), 520–526. https://doi.org/10.1002/gps.2559

Allaz, A.-F., & Cedraschi, C. (2015). *Emotional aspects of chronic pain*. In G. Pickering & S. Gibson (Eds.), *Pain, Emotion and Cognition: A Complex Nexus* (pp. 21–34). New York, NY: Springer.

Amariglio, R. E., Townsend, M. K., Grodstein, F., Sperling, R. A, & Rentz, D. M. (2011). Specific subjective memory complaints in older persons may indicate poor cognitive function. *Journal of the American Geriatrics Society, 59*(9), 1612–1617. https://doi.org/10.1111/j.1532-5415.2011.03543.x

Binder, L. M., Iverson, G. L., & Brooks, B. L. (2009). To err is human: "Abnormal" neuropsychological scores and variability are common in healthy adults. *Archives of Clinical Neuropsychology, 24*(1), 31–46. https://doi.org/10.1093/arclin/acn001

Buckley, R. F., Villemagne, V. L., Masters, C. L., Ellis, K. A., Rowe, C. C., Johnson, K., … Amariglio, R. (2016). A conceptualization of the utility of subjective cognitive decline in clinical trials of preclinical Alzheimer's disease. *Journal of Molecular Neuroscience, 60*(3), 354–361. https://doi.org/10.1007/s12031-016-0810-z

Buckley, R. F., Saling, M. M., Frommann, I., Wolfsgruber, S., & Wagner, M. (2015). Subjective cognitive decline from a phenomenological perspective: A review of the qualitative literature. *Journal of Alzheimer's Disease, 48*(Suppl 1), S125–S140. https://doi.org/10.3233/JAD-150095

Canadian Institutes of Health Research. (2013). Information about Alzheimer's and related dementias. Retrieved from http://www.cihr-irsc.gc.ca/e/45554.html

Chen, K.-L., Sun, Y.-M., Zhou, Y., Zhao, Q.-H., Ding, D., & Guo, Q.-H. (2016). Associations between APOE polymorphisms and seven diseases with cognitive impairment including Alzheimer's disease, frontotemporal dementia, and dementia with Lewy bodies in southeast China. *Psychiatric Genetics*, *26*(3), 124–131. https://doi.org/10.1097/YPG.0000000000000126

Cherbuin, N., Sargent-Cox, K., Easteal, S., Sachdev, P., & Anstey, K. J. (2015). Hippocampal atrophy is associated with subjective memory decline: The PATH Through Life Study. *American Journal of Geriatric Psychiatry*, *23*(5), 546–556. https://doi.org/10.1016/j.jagp.2014.07.009

Comijs, H. C., Deeg, D. J. H., Dik, M. G., Twisk, J. W. R., & Jonker, C. (2002). Memory complaints; the association with psycho-affective and health problems and the role of personality characteristics. A 6-year follow-up study. *Journal of Affective Disorders*, *72*(2), 157–165. https://doi.org/10.1016/S0165-0327(01)00453-0

Cooper, C., Bebbington, P., Lindesay, J., Meltzer, H., McManus, S., Jenkins, R., & Livingston, G. (2011). The meaning of reporting forgetfulness: A cross-sectional study of adults in the English 2007 Adult Psychiatric Morbidity Survey. *Age and Ageing*, *40*(6), 711–717. https://doi.org/10.1093/ageing/afr121

Creswell, J. W., & Poth, C. N. (2017). *Qualitative Inquiry and Research Design. Choosing Among Five Approaches*. Thousand Oaks, CA: SAGE.

Derouesné, C., Lacomblez, L., Thibault, S., & LePoncin, M. (1999). Memory complaints in young and elderly subjects. *International Journal of Geriatric Psychiatry*, *14*(4), 291–301. https://doi.org/10.1002/(SICI)1099-1166(199904)14:4<291::AID-GPS902>3.0.CO;2-7

Dhilla Albers, A., Asafu-Adjei, J., Delaney, M. K., Kelly, K. E., Gomez-Isla, T., Blacker, D., …

Albers, M. W. (2016). Episodic memory of odors stratifies Alzheimer biomarkers in normal

elderly. *Annals of Neurology, 80*(6), 846–857. https://doi.org/10.1002/ana.24792

Dux, M. C., Woodard, J. L., Calamari, J. E., Messina, M., Arora, S., Chik, H., & Pontarelli, N.

(2008). The moderating role of negative affect on objective verbal memory performance and

subjective memory complaints in healthy older adults. *Journal of the International

Neuropsychological Society: JINS, 14*(2), 327–336.

https://doi.org/10.1017/S1355617708080363

Edmonds, E. C., Delano-Wood, L., Galasko, D. R., Salmon, D. P., & Bondi, M. W. (2015).

Subtle cognitive decline and biomarker staging in preclinical Alzheimer's disease. *Journal

of Alzheimer's Disease, 47*(1), 231–242. https://doi.org/10.3233/JAD-150128

Edmonds, E. C., McDonald, C. R., Marshall, A., Thomas, K. R., Eppig, J., Weigand, A. J., …

Bondi, M. W. (2019). Early versus late MCI: Improved MCI staging using a

neuropsychological approach. *Alzheimer's and Dementia, 15*(5), 699–708.

https://doi.org/10.1016/j.jalz.2018.12.009

Farrer, L. A., Cupples, A. L., Kukull, W. a, Mayeux, R., Myers, R. H., Pericak-vance, M. a, …

van Duijn, C. M. (1997). Effects of age , sex , and ethnicity on the association between

apolipoprotein E genotype and Alzheimer disease. *JAMA: The Journal of the American

Medical Association, 278*, 1349–1356. https://doi.org/10.1001/jama.1997.03550160069041

Fonseca, J. A. S., Ducksbury, R., Rodda, J., Whitfield, T., Nagaraj, C., Suresh, K., … Walker, Z.

(2015). Factors that predict cognitive decline in patients with subjective cognitive

impairment. *International Psychogeriatrics/IPA, 27*(10), 1671–1677.

https://doi.org/10.1017/S1041610215000356

Fortea, J., Sala-Llonch, R., Bartrés-Faz, D., Lladó, A., Solé-Padullés, C., Bosch, B., … Rami, L.

(2011). Cognitively preserved subjects with transitional cerebrospinal fluid β-amyloid 1-42 values have thicker cortex in Alzheimer's disease vulnerable areas. *Biological Psychiatry, 70*(2), 183–190. https://doi.org/10.1016/j.biopsych.2011.02.017

Gibson, S. J. (2015). The pain, emotion and cognition nexus in older persons and in dementia. In G. Pickering & S. Gibson (Eds.), *Pain, Emotion and Cognition: A Complex Nexus* (pp. 231–247). New York, NY: Springer.

Goesling, J., Clauw, D. J., & Hassett, A. L. (2013). Pain and depression: An integrative review of neurobiological and psychological factors. *Current Psychiatry Reports, 15*(12), 421. https://doi.org/10.1007/s11920-013-0421-0

Hall, A., Mattila, J., Koikkalainen, J., Lötjonen, J., Wolz, R., Scheltens, P., … Soininen, H. (2015). Predicting progression from cognitive impairment to Alzheimer's disease with the Disease State Index. *Current Alzheimer Research, 12*(1), 69–79. https://doi.org/10.2174/1567205012666141218123829

Imtiaz, B., Tolppanen, A. M., Kivipelto, M., & Soininen, H. (2014). Future directions in Alzheimer's disease from risk factors to prevention. *Biochemical Pharmacology, 88*(4), 661–670. https://doi.org/10.1016/j.bcp.2014.01.003

Jack, C. R., Bennett, D. A., Blennow, K., Carrillo, M. C., Dunn, B., Haeberlein, S. B., … Silverberg, N. (2018). NIA-AA Research Framework: Toward a biological definition of Alzheimer's disease. *Alzheimer's and Dementia, 14*(4), 535–562. https://doi.org/10.1016/j.jalz.2018.02.018

Jessen, F., Amariglio, R. E., Buckley, R. F., van der Flier, W. M., Han, Y., Molinuevo, J. L., … Wagner, M. (2020). The characterisation of subjective cognitive decline. *The Lancet Neurology, 19*(3), 271–278. https://doi.org/10.1016/S1474-4422(19)30368-0

Jessen, F., Amariglio, R. E., Van Boxtel, M., Breteler, M., Ceccaldi, M., Chételat, G., …

Wagner, M. (2014). A conceptual framework for research on subjective cognitive decline in

preclinical Alzheimer's disease. *Alzheimer's and Dementia, 10*(6), 844–852.

https://doi.org/10.1016/j.jalz.2014.01.001

Jessen, F., Wiese, B., Bachmann, C., Eifflaender-Gorfer, S., Haller, F., Kölsch, H., … Bickel, H.

(2010). Prediction of dementia by subjective memory impairment effects of severity and

temporal association with cognitive impairment. *Archives of General Psychiatry, 67*(4),

414–422. https://doi.org/10.1001/archgenpsychiatry.2010.30

Jessen, F., Wiese, B., Cvetanovska, G., Fuchs, A., Kaduszkiewicz, H., Kölsch, H., … Bickel, H.

(2007). Patterns of subjective memory impairment in the elderly: Association with memory

performance. *Psychological Medicine, 37*(12), 1753–1762.

https://doi.org/10.1017/S0033291707001122

Jessen, F., Wolfsgruber, S., Wiese, B., Bickel, H., Mösch, E., Kaduszkiewicz, H., … Wagner, M.

(2014). AD dementia risk in late MCI, in early MCI, and in subjective memory impairment.

Alzheimer's and Dementia, 10(1), 76–83. https://doi.org/10.1016/j.jalz.2012.09.017

Jiang, S., Tang, L., Zhao, N., Yang, W., Qiu, Y., & Chen, H. Z. (2016). A systems view of the

differences between APOE ε4 carriers and non-carriers in Alzheimer's disease. *Frontiers in

Aging Neuroscience, 8*, 171. https://doi.org/10.3389/fnagi.2016.00171

Jonker, C., Geerlings, M. I., & Schmand, B. (2000). Are memory complaints predictive for

dementia?. A review of clinical and population-based studies. *International Journal of

Geriatric Psychiatry, 15*(11), 983–991. https://doi.org/10.1002/1099-

1166(200011)15:11<983::aid-gps238>3.0.co;2-5

Kielb, S., Rogalski, E., Weintraub, S., & Rademaker, A. (2017). Objective features of subjective

cognitive decline in a United States national database. *Alzheimer's and Dementia, 13*(12),

1337–1344. https://doi.org/10.1016/j.jalz.2017.04.008

Krell-Roesch, J., Woodruff, B. K., Acosta, J. I., Locke, D. E., Hentz, J. G., Stonnington, C. M.,

    … Geda, Y. E. (2015). APOE ε4 genotype and the risk for subjective cognitive impairment

    in elderly persons. *The Journal of Neuropsychiatry and Clinical Neurosciences, 27*(4), 322–

    325. https://doi.org/10.1176/appi.neuropsych.14100268

Lista, S., Molinuevo, J. L., Cavedo, E., Rami, L., Amouyel, P., Teipel, S. J., … Hampel, H.

    (2015). Evolving evidence for the value of neuroimaging methods and biological markers in

    subjects categorized with subjective cognitive decline. *Journal of Alzheimer's Disease,*

    48(S1), S171–S191. https://doi.org/10.3233/JAD-150202

Liu, Y., Tan, L., Wang, H.-F., Liu, Y., Hao, X.-K., Tan, C.-C., … Alzheimer's Disease

    Neuroimaging Initiative. (2016). Multiple effect of APOE genotype on clinical and

    neuroimaging biomarkers across Alzheimer's disease spectrum. *Molecular Neurobiology,*

    53(7), 4539–4547. https://doi.org/10.1007/s12035-015-9388-7

Mata, I. F., Leverenz, J. B., Weintraub, D., Trojanowski, J. Q., Hurtig, H. I., Van Deerlin, V. M.,

    … Zabetian, C. P. (2014). APOE, MAPT, and SNCA genes and cognitive performance in

    Parkinson disease. *JAMA Neurology, 71*(11), 1405–1412.

    https://doi.org/10.1001/jamaneurol.2014.1455

Mattsson, N., Insel, P. S., Donohue, M., Landau, S., Jagust, W. J., Shaw, L. M., … Weiner, M.

    W. (2015). Independent information from cerebrospinal fluid amyloid-β and florbetapir

    imaging in Alzheimer's disease. *Brain, 138*(3), 772–783.

    https://doi.org/10.1093/brain/awu367

Molinuevo, J. L., Rabin, L. A., Amariglio, R., Buckley, R., Dubois, B., Ellis, K. A., … Jessen, F.

    (2017). Implementation of subjective cognitive decline criteria in research studies.

Alzheimer's and Dementia, 13(3), 296–311. https://doi.org/10.1016/j.jalz.2016.09.012

Nikolai, T., Bezdicek, O., Markova, H., Stepankova, H., Michalec, J., Kopecek, M., … Vyhnalek, M. (2018). Semantic verbal fluency impairment is detectable in patients with subjective cognitive decline. *Applied Neuropsychology:Adult, 25*(5), 448–457. https://doi.org/10.1080/23279095.2017.1326047

Pink, A., Stokin, G. B., Bartley, M. M., Roberts, R. O., Sochor, O., Machulda, M. M., … Geda, Y. E. (2015). Neuropsychiatric symptoms, APOE ε4, and the risk of incident dementia: A population-based study. *Neurology, 84*(9), 935–943. https://doi.org/10.1212/WNL.0000000000001307

Prestia, A., Caroli, A., Wade, S. K., van der Flier, W. M., Ossenkoppele, R., Van Berckel, B., … Frisoni, G. B. (2015). Prediction of AD dementia by biomarkers following the NIA-AA and IWG diagnostic criteria in MCI patients from three European memory clinics. *Neuropsychology Review, 11*(10), 1191–1201. https://doi.org/10.1016/j.jalz.2014.12.001

Rabin, L. A., Smart, C. M., Crane, P. K., Amariglio, R. E., Berman, L. M., Boada, M., … Sikkes, S. A. M. (2015). Subjective cognitive decline in older adults: An overview of self-report measures used across 19 international research studies. *Journal of Alzheimer's Disease, 48*(S1), S63–S86. https://doi.org/10.3233/JAD-150154

Reisberg, B., Shulman, M. B., Torossian, C., Leng, L., & Zhu, W. (2010). Outcome over seven years of healthy adults with and without subjective cognitive impairment. *Neuropsychology Review, 6*(1), 11–24. https://doi.org/10.1016/j.jalz.2009.10.002

Risacher, S. L., Kim, S., Nho, K., Foroud, T., Shen, L., Petersen, R. C., … Alzheimer's Disease Neuroimaging Initiative (ADNI). (2015). APOE effect on Alzheimer's disease biomarkers in older adults with significant memory concern. *Alzheimer's and Dementia, 11*(12), 1417–

1429. https://doi.org/10.1016/j.jalz.2015.03.003

Sierra-Rio, A., Balasa, M., Olives, J., Antonell, A., Iranzo, A., Castellví, M., … Molinuevo, J. L. (2016). Cerebrospinal fluid biomarkers predict clinical evolution in patients with subjective cognitive decline and mild cognitive impairment. *Neurodegenerative Diseases, 16*(1–2), 69–76. https://doi.org/10.1159/000439258

Slavin, M. J., Brodaty, H., Kochan, N. A., Crawford, J. D., Trollor, J. N., Draper, B., & Sachdev, P. S. (2010). Prevalence and predictors of "subjective cognitive complaints" in the Sydney Memory and Ageing Study. *American Journal of Geriatric Psychiatry, 18*(8), 701–710. https://doi.org/10.1097/JGP.0b013e3181df49fb

Smart, C. M., Karr, J. E., Areshenkoff, C. N., Rabin, L. A., Hudon, C., Gates, N., … Wesselman, L. (2017). Non-Pharmacologic interventions for older adults with subjective cognitive decline: Systematic review, meta-analysis, and preliminary recommendations.

Sperling, R. A., Aisen, P. S., Beckett, L. A., Bennett, D. A., Craft, S., Fagan, A. M., … Phelps, C. H. (2011). Toward defining the preclinical stages of Alzheimer's disease: Recommendations from the National Institute on Aging-Alzheimer's Association workgroups on diagnostic guidelines for Alzheimer's disease. *Alzheimer's and Dementia, 7*(3), 280–292. https://doi.org/10.1016/j.jalz.2011.03.003

Stewart, R., Russ, C., Richards, M., Brayne, C., Lovestone, S., & Mann, A. (2001). Depression, APOE genotype and subjective memory impairment: A cross-sectional study in an African-Caribbean population. *Psychological Medicine, 31*(3), 431–440.

Stewart, R., Godin, O., Crivello, F., Maillard, P., Mazoyer, B., Tzourio, C., & Dufouil, C. (2011). Longitudinal neuroimaging correlates of subjective memory impairment: 4-year prospective community study. *British Journal of Psychiatry, 198*(3), 199–205. https://doi.org/10.1192/bjp.bp.110.078683

Striepens, N., Scheef, L., Wind, A., Popp, J., Spottke, A., Cooper-Mahkorn, D., … Jessen, F.

    (2010). Volume loss of the medial temporal lobe structures in subjective memory

    impairment. *Dementia and Geriatric Cognitive Disorders, 29*(1), 75–81.

    https://doi.org/10.1159/000264630

Tuokko, H. A., & Smart, C. M. (2018). *Neuropsychology of cognitive decline: A developmental*

    approach to assessment and intervention. New York, NY: Guilford Press.

Verlinden, V. J. A., van der Geest, J. N., de Bruijn, R. F. A. G., Hofman, A., Koudstaal, P. J., &

    Ikram, M. A. (2017). Trajectories of decline in cognition and daily functioning in preclinical

    dementia. *Alzheimer's and Dementia, 12*(2), 1–10. https://doi.org/10.1016/j.jalz.2015.08.001

Wolfsgruber, S., Kleineidam, L., Wagner, M., Mösch, E., Bickel, H., Lühmann, D., … Jessen, F.

    (2016). Differential risk of incident Alzheimer's disease dementia in stable versus unstable

    patterns of subjective cognitive decline. *Journal of Alzheimer's Disease, 54*(3), 1135–1146.

    https://doi.org/10.3233/JAD-160407

Introduction

A recent report by the U.S. Census Bureau and National Institute on Aging predicts that, by 2020, for the first time the world population of people over 65 years will surpass the number of children born, and that older adults may comprise as much as 16% of the world's population by 2050 [1]. This demographic shift is due in part to decreasing fertility rates, but also increased longevity made possible by health care advances and a generally higher standard of living. Although the thriving of older adults may be hailed as a triumph in many respects, disorders of aging, such as all-cause dementia, become an increasingly salient concern as the number of adults living into late life increases. For instance, it is projected that as many as 14 million older adults in the United States may develop Alzheimer's disease (AD), the leading cause of dementia, by 2050 [2]. In light of this, much research has been dedicated to identifying early indicators of pathological aging, with particular emphasis on understanding predictors of non-normative cognitive decline [3,4].

As our understanding of pathological aging has grown, an increasing number of impairing prodromal conditions, such as mild cognitive impairment (MCI), have been identified; however, recent studies have suggested that subjective cognitive decline (SCD) may precede even these as the earliest indication of incipient neuropathology [5]. SCD is generally defined as self- and/or informant-perceived decline in cognitive function in spite of performance within normal limits on standardized neuropsychological tests [6]. Historically, older adults with SCD may have largely been regarded as the "worried well" given the lack of objective evidence of impairment. However, more recent evidence suggests that, for as many as 60% of individuals with SCD, these self-perceived changes may indeed herald cognitive decline to dementia [7]. Thus, given that early detection of persons at risk is widely considered the key to instituting effective preventive strategies for cognitive decline and dementia, understanding SCD is of obvious import to clinicians and researchers.

Since AD is the most prevalent form of dementia, it may be unsurprising that the majority of SCD research has been aimed at characterizing SCD as a potential prodromal form of AD. This goal has been somewhat achieved thanks to both longitudinal [8,9] and cross-sectional studies [10,11] indicating that those with SCD evidence a higher number of known AD biomarkers than healthy controls and, consequently, that they may be at higher risk of developing AD in future. Despite this traditional AD focus, however, there is evidence to suggest that SCD may confer a more general risk of developing other reversible [12] and non-reversible [13,14] dementing conditions as well. Nevertheless, this review will focus exclusively on SCD as a form of preclinical AD in light of the SCD-Initiative Working Group's AD-oriented definition of SCD [15,16] and the surfeit of available research committed to explicating this specific relationship.

To better elucidate the relationship between SCD and later cognitive decline, numerous efforts have been made to identify optimally sensitive self-report measures and neuropsychological predictors of later decline [17,18]; however, consensus has remained elusive [18–20]. A particular difficulty for clinical neuropsychologists has been that cognitive and functional measures typically used to make a clinical diagnosis appear relatively insensitive at the very earliest, asymptomatic stages of cognitive decline [6]. Currently, the determination of SCD rests largely on self-report; however, most of the measures currently used are designed for populations other than SCD and, thus, may lack sensitivity, specificity, and/or construct validity for this population [18]. Further, the determination of cognitive impairment often relies on a binary classification scheme (i.e., either impaired vs. unimpaired), which may be ill-suited for identifying subtle decrements in those whose neuropsychological functioning is average by definition [6] but above-average more typically [19].

This is particularly relevant given the evidence that persons with higher education who have SCD seem to be at greater risk of decline than those with lower education [21].

In sum, the mixed outcomes for those with SCD, as well as the seeming insensitivity of neuropsychological measures to corroborate self-reported cognitive disturbances, raises questions about how to distinguish those aging normally from those who are legitimately experiencing pathological, albeit subtle, cognitive change.

Subjective Cognitive Decline and the APOE ε4 Genotype

Given the insufficiency of current self-report and neuropsychological approaches to resolve this question, a parallel line of research has probed the value of various biomarkers, any of a number of biological/physiological correlates of known pathology, for predicting later cognitive decline. The growing reliance on biomarker data for diagnosis may be illustrated best by the recently updated NIA-AA research framework, which argues that AD would be better defined by distinct neuropathology and a specific biomarker profile (i.e., evidence of Aβ deposition paired with increased deposition of paired helical filament tau) than cognitive symptoms [22]. Despite this proposed departure from symptom-based diagnosis, however, this framework may still be largely predicated on the presence of neuropathological biomarkers among clinical samples with at least some degree of objective impairment (i.e., AD, MCI). It is less clear how a purely biomarker-led approach to AD diagnosis may be leveraged in a clinical setting where individuals demonstrate a complete lack of apparent concerns or cognitive symptoms. Thus, as with neuropsychological approaches, relatively sound guidelines appear to have been established for the determination of neurodegenerative conditions, but these may be most relevant *once impairment is apparent.*

One of the most robust findings in recent years has been that the presence of the ε4 variant of the apolipoprotein E (APOE ε4) imparts a genetic risk for the development of cognitive impairment, specifically that related to AD and vascular dementia [23–29]. The APOE gene is integrally involved in cholesterol metabolism and the maintenance of cholesterol homeostasis in the brain [30]. APOE ε4 is relatively common among the general population, though its prevalence differs across geographic and ethnic lines. APOE ε4 carriers are most common in Oceania (62.44%), and Northern Europe (61.25%), and lowest in Asia (41.88%), and Southern/Mediterranean Europe (40.45%) [31]. Despite – or perhaps, because of – the wide distribution of APOE ε4, the specific risk conferred to carriers has remained unclear. APOE ε4 carriers have been estimated to be 2.2 [32] to 6.2 [33] times more likely to develop MCI than non-carriers. Single allele carriers are estimated to have a 2.6 to 3.2 times greater risk of developing AD, while double allele carriers are estimated to be approximately 15 times more likely than the general population to develop AD [34]. APOE ε4 carriers with cognitive impairment or MCI have also been shown to have increased risk of AD conversion ranging from 4.1 [32] to 25 times that of non-carriers [35]. This would seem supported by a large-scale meta-analysis of case-controlled studies that found significantly higher frequency of APOE ε4 among AD samples (38% overall) compared to healthy controls (14% overall) [36]. Given the relatively well-understood link to AD-consistent pathology, APOE ε4 data may provide crucial insight into risk for cognitive decline among those with SCD.

Until relatively recently, SCD was not well characterized and, consequently, was not amenable to rigorous study. To better understand and codify this clinical condition, the SCD-Initiative (SCD-I) working group was established [15]. This not only allowed for more concerted efforts to understand and characterize SCD, but also led to the development of comprehensive guidelines for studying SCD [16]. Particularly notable about the SCD-I's framework for classifying SCD is the special designation of SCD *Plus*, additional SCD criteria associated with the highest risk of later conversion to AD [15]. Along with recommendations to attend to the level of individuals' concern about their perceived deficits, their age, and time since onset of perceived deficits, the SCD *Plus* guidelines explicitly encourage the collection of biomarker data, including APOE ε4 genotype data, to supplement neuropsychological test scores and self- and informant reports. This is congruent with current NIA preclinical AD criteria, which stipulates the use of biomarker data to determine the presence of AD-consistent pathophysiological processes in those with subtle or absent observable symptoms [22].

Since the establishment of the SCD-I and their classification framework, substantially more work has been dedicated to exploring the convergent features of SCD and neurodegenerative conditions, like AD [5,16]. Accordingly, literature focused specifically on investigating the presence and meaning of dementia-risk biomarkers in SCD has burgeoned as well [37]. Interest in the APOE ε4 biomarker's role in SCD specifically has dominated the field, likely due to its reliably demonstrated relationship with pathological cognitive decline [23,24] and its quick, non-invasive, and relatively low-cost method of collection compared to other biomarkers such as amyloid-β or tau [38]. In light of this bloom in research and the rapid accumulation of novel information regarding the relationship between SCD and APOE ε4, a systematic review of the field is not only prudent but also necessary to consolidate our understanding of SCD and its relationship to pathological cognitive decline. Understanding the cross-sectional and longitudinal relationships between SCD and APOE ε4 might allow for greater quantification of risk of cognitive decline and dementia when individuals prospectively present with SCD.

Objectives of the Current Review

Given the documented relationships between APOE ε4 and subsequent decline to AD, and in light of the recent proliferation of research on the role of APOE ε4 in the relationship between SCD and AD, the current review is especially timely. However, in addition to the academic value presented by this work, the current review may also be particularly beneficial to clinicians. The ambiguous relationship between SCD and AD has posed a considerable challenge for clinical neuropsychologists in particular who, tasked with assessing the veracity and clinical significance of cognitive complaints, are frequently hampered in their efforts by a lack of objective cognitive data on which to base a clinical opinion. Consequently, current practice is resigned to adopting an inefficient wait-and-see approach to determine whether any given case of SCD is in fact an augur of pathological cognitive decline to come. Due to this lack of reliable risk assessment, aggressive early intervention remains difficult to justify to medical service providers and potentially unethical to recommend to patients (i.e., due to the potential for eliciting undue concern and distress) [39], despite the fact that emerging evidence suggests that early intervention could have beneficial effects on cognitive function in persons with SCD [40].

A primary aim of this review was to evaluate whether otherwise healthy individuals with SCD are more likely than those without SCD to have at least one APOE ε4 allele. Moreover, as the association of APOE ε4 with AD has been well-established for some time, another goal of this review is to evaluate the evidence that those with SCD and at least one APOE ε4 allele are more disposed to the development of AD than those either without SCD or with SCD but without any APOE ε4 alleles. An overarching objective was that this review would enable clinicians and clinical researchers to better determine the practicality of employing APOE ε4 genetic testing in practice as a means to identify risk of objective cognitive decline in those presenting with SCD.

Methods

Eligibility Criteria

Only English-language, peer-reviewed, human studies with available full-text articles were considered eligible for inclusion. As this review is concerned with the relationship between SCD and APOE ε4, eligible studies were those that included samples of individuals identified as having SCD or conceptually equivalent conditions who were absent of objective impairment as per standardized test data [15]. It should be noted that, since this is the first systematic review of SCD conversion risk factors undertaken since the establishment of the SCD-Initiative criteria [15], the exact classification of participants in some prior studies may be uncertain. As the construct of SCD is categorical [15], studies that addressed complaints as a continuous variable were excluded. The specific terminology used in each included study is summarized in Table 1. In addition to SCD-related criteria, eligible studies were also required to include information pertaining to either the incidence of APOE ε4 genotype among those with SCD relative to other groups, or the impact of APOE ε4 status on symptoms and/or outcomes for those with SCD. The age of included study samples was limited to 55 years and older. The lower threshold of 55 years was selected to account for the approximate 15-year timeframe to AD conversion that has been previously discussed [41] and to align with evidence that APOE ε4 confers greatest risk of cognitive decline beginning at approximately age 55 years [42,43]. Studies with a lower minimum age were included if they provided age-stratified data with a distinct 55+ age group. No restrictions were placed on sample type, though this was accounted for (Table 2). Given the fledgling state of the field, it was considered both unnecessary and unduly limiting to place restrictions on year of publication.

Search Strategy

PubMed and EBSCOhost databases, including Cochrane Central Register of Controlled Trials, Medline with Full Text, CINAHL Complete, and PsycINFO databases were searched using a combination of relevant keywords agreed upon by the authors (see appendix A for search terms in full). The search protocol was executed separately on the same day (April 29, 2018) by each of the authors to promote reliability. Following an initial screen to exclude ineligible articles and duplicates, the suitability of each article was independently adjudicated by two of the authors (two of JIA, CMS, JRG). Where there was disagreement between the initial raters, the third author's rating determined whether a given study was included.

Outcome Measures

Firstly, this review sought to provide information regarding the degree to which those individuals with SCD carry the APOE ε4 genotype relative to those without SCD. A statistical analysis was performed to determine the prevalence of APOE ε4 in SCD samples relative to healthy controls and objectively impaired samples across studies. Statistical analysis of the impact of SCD classification method (e.g., self-report vs. informant report, questionnaire vs. single question) was not performed as there was insufficient power to perform any meaningful analysis between cohorts. An additional outcome of interest was the extent to which those with SCD and the APOE ε4 genotype are at greater risk for later AD.

Data Analysis and Synthesis

For each study, the term/construct of interest (e.g., SCD, subjective memory impairment, subjective cognitive complaints), mean sample age and composition, and sample type are provided alongside ratings of methodological strength. Results across studies are discussed in terms of consistencies and inconsistencies within the sample of included studies, as well as in relation to the literature at large. Analysis of the prevalence of APOE ε4 across diagnostic categories (e.g., SCD, MCI, AD) was calculated using IBM SPSS Statistics software version 22.

Results

Systematic Review

The initial search supplied 461 articles (CINAHL Complete 81; Cochrane Central Register of Controlled Trials 28; MEDLINE with Full Text 172; PsycINFO 119; PubMed 61). Following manual removal of duplicates and ostensibly irrelevant entries (e.g., those that controlled for APOE genotype, reviews and other secondary sources), an initial sample of 115 articles was identified for more in-depth review and vetting. Each of these articles was assigned to two authors (two of JIA, CMS, or JRG) who independently evaluated each entry for its suitability based on demographic criteria and relevance to the topic of interest. Where there was disagreement between the initial raters ($n = 12$ articles), the third author evaluated the discrepancy and made the final decision. The majority of exclusions were due to an undefined SCD group (e.g., lack of discrimination between those with SCD and MCI; 38 articles) or violation of the 55 years or older criteria (31 articles). This process is summarized in Figure 1. A list of the articles excluded from this review is provided in the supplementary materials. A sample of 36 articles published between 2001 and 2018 were included in the final review.

Study Design and Sample Type

With few exceptions, the included studies concentrated on elucidating cross-sectional relationships between APOE status and SCD. Though valuable, this cross-sectional focus introduces interpretive complications. Since the essential value of APOE ε4 as a biomarker is its predictive value for future pathological cognitive decline, longitudinal designs may provide more directly relevant information. Further, given the heterogeneity in SCD sample definition and eligibility criteria across studies (Table 1; Table S1 in Supplemental Materials), it is likely that persons with SCD data represent a more diverse range of clinical presentations and etiologies than other defined clinical groups (i.e., MCI, AD). This asymmetric variability is likely to impact cross-sectional between-group findings more than longitudinal within-group results. With this in mind, cross-sectional and longitudinal findings have been presented separately where applicable in the sections below.

An additional caveat relates to sample type. There is evidence to suggest that individuals recruited from memory clinics and other medical settings may differ in important ways from those recruited from the community. For instance, individuals presenting to clinics may experience a greater degree of distress related to SCD than those who do not. Indeed, Perrotin et al. demonstrated that subclinical depressive symptoms and hippocampal atrophy are specifically associated with medically help seeking among those with SCD [44]. Conversely, there is concern that samples derived from memory clinics or other specialized settings may misrepresent the full scope of SCD-related symptoms (e.g., memory clinics may preferentially assess and report memory symptoms). There was an insufficient number of community/clinical studies to divide the results in any meaningful way by sample type; however, sample type has been clarified as necessary throughout the following sections.

Prevalence of APOE ε4 in SCD

Of the 36 articles in the systematic review, 27 provided clear data regarding the prevalence of APOE ε4 in their respective SCD samples compared to other identified groups (e.g., healthy controls, MCI). Twenty-six articles provided comparison data for healthy control samples, while 15 provided comparison data for MCI samples and 7 provided comparison data for diagnosed/probable AD. A Freeman-Tukey arcsine transformation was applied to the APOE ε4-positive frequency values provided by each study [45]. A univariate ANOVA was conducted to determine whether there was a significant difference in the prevalence of the APOE ε4 allele among individuals with SCD relative to healthy controls and samples with objective cognitive impairment (i.e., MCI and diagnosed/probable AD). Sample type (i.e., community vs. clinic) was included as a covariate and the analysis was weighted according to sample size per diagnostic group per study (i.e., HC, SCD, MCI, AD). There was a significant main effect of diagnosis on APOE ε4 allele frequency ($F = 23.06$, $p < .001$, partial $\eta^2 = .52$). Post-hoc pairwise comparisons indicated no significant difference in APOE ε4 frequency between SCD ($M = 28.60\%$) and healthy controls ($M = 24.48\%$; $p = .29$), but significantly lower APOE ε4 frequency in SCD relative to MCI ($M = 46.98\%$, $p = .001$) and diagnosed or probable AD ($M = 78.44\%$, $p < .001$). Comparing the mean frequency of APOE ε4 across groups, the proportional representation of APOE ε4 carrier status increased with degree of objective impairment (i.e., healthy controls/SCD < MCI < AD). Sample type did not have a significant main effect on the prevalence of APOE ε4 ($F = 3.17, p = .08$).

Neurobiological Changes

Cross-sectional results. Four studies ($n = 3$ clinic; $n = 1$ mixed sample) undertook cross-sectional investigations of potential neurobiological differences in APOE ε4-carrying individuals with SCD relative to other groups. Striepens and coworkers' manual tracing protocol found that APOE ε4-positive individuals with SCD had significantly smaller left hippocampi ($p = .03$) [46] than healthy controls. Lee et al.'s [47] voxel-based morphometry approach, on the other hand, indicated that APOE ε4-positive individuals with SCD were found to have significantly more gray matter atrophy in the inferior temporal gyrus, inferior parietal lobe, anterior cingulum, middle frontal gyrus, and precentral gyrus ($p < .001$) compared to non-carriers with SCD. In addition to deterioration in cortical gray matter, there is some evidence that APOE ε4-positive individuals with SCD may experience loss of white matter integrity as well. Lee and coworkers [47] found significantly lower fractional anisotropy (a DTI marker for white matter disruption; $p < .05$) in the anterior corona radiata and the splenium of the corpus callosum among APOE ε4 carriers with SCD. This pattern of white matter disruption was reported to simulate AD-type pathology in quality if not quantity. In contrast, neither SCD [48] nor APOE status were found to be linked to the presence of white matter hyperintensities among clinical or mixed clinical/community samples [47,49].

Longitudinal results. The two community-based longitudinal studies of neurobiological change included in this review provided mixed results. Stewart and coworkers [50] found that the presence of SCD was linked to significant decreases in hippocampal volume ($p = .005$) relative to healthy controls. At four-year follow up, those with memory complaints showed a significant volume change in cerebrospinal fluid (CSF; ($p = .002$), subcortical white matter ($p = .022$), the hippocampi ($p < .012$), and gray matter ($p < .001$). Likewise, Cherbuin and team [51] found that individuals with newly developed SCD in the approximate four-year span between time 1 and time 2 testing exhibited significantly smaller right hippocampal volumes and a significantly greater degree of bilateral hippocampal atrophy relative to healthy controls. Those with chronic SCD experienced greater right hippocampal atrophy than those with newly developed SCD and healthy controls. Despite general consensus regarding the conferred risk of SCD status, however, there was a marked discrepancy between the studies regarding the role of APOE ε4 status. Where Stewart and colleagues [50] found that the association between SCD and the aforementioned neurobiological changes was significantly stronger among APOE ε4 carriers, Cherbuin and coworkers found no such relationship [51].

Amyloid Burden

Six cross-sectional studies ($n = 1$ clinic; $n = 5$ mixed, community sample) directly addressed the interaction between APOE ε4 and amyloid burden in persons with SCD. Several suggest that SCD and APOE ε4 genotype confer independent and additive risk of amyloid deposition, a key characteristic of Alzheimer's-type pathology. An imaging study by Risacher and colleagues [52] found that individuals presenting to clinic with APOE ε4 and SCD together exhibited more amyloid deposition in bilateral cingulate, frontal, temporal, and parietal lobar regions than those with SCD but no APOE ε4. In fact, along with APOE ε4-positive individuals with early MCI, APOE ε4-positive individuals with SCD had greater amyloid deposition in all regions of interest compared to APOE ε4-negative individuals. Inversely, several community studies have found that individuals with SCD and verified high amyloid burden were significantly more likely to carry the APOE ε4 allele [53–55]. The additive risk of SCD and APOE ε4 genotype on amyloid burden has also been borne out by a post-mortem autopsy study that found APOE ε4 carriers with reported SCD at the time of death exhibited significantly greater amyloid deposition ($p = .003$) [56]. Despite this body of evidence, the relationship between SCD, APOE ε4, and amyloid burden may not be equilateral. Zwan and colleagues [57] identified APOE ε4 ($p < .05$) and SCD ($p < .05$) as independent risk factors for increased amyloid burden among a community sample; however, further investigation indicated that the presence of SCD conferred increased risk exclusively in APOE ε4 carriers ($p = .002$). Rowe and coworkers [58] found a similar interaction ($p < .001$) in their community sample. In both cases, the relationship between SCD and amyloid burden was mediated by APOE ε4-positive status. With regard to amyloid burden, there was no clear difference between the findings of studies using community or clinical samples.

Conversion to Objective Impairment and/or Dementia

Given that meaningful assessment of dementia conversion requires monitoring over time and follow up at multiple time points, the following section exclusively features data from longitudinal investigations. Both Hong et al. [59] and Jessen et al. [60] have found APOE ε4 status to be among the strongest predictors for conversion from SCD to an objectively cognitively impaired state among individuals presenting to clinics ($p < .02$ and $p < .001$, respectively). Dik and coworkers' community study [8] supports this contention and provides additional evidence of an interaction effect between APOE ε4 status and SCD. They found that, relative to APOE ε4-negative healthy controls, MMSE scores for APOE ε4-negative individuals with SCD and APOE ε4-positive controls declined significantly more over six years (1.2 points vs. 0.8 points and 1.4 points vs. 0.8 points, respectively). Moreover, APOE ε4 carriers with SCD showed additive risk beyond that represented by either SCD or APOE ε4 alone (decrease of 1.7 points vs. 0.8 points). Supporting this interaction, Kryscio and colleagues' [56] post-mortem examination of dementia course and survivorship among community-dwelling older adults found that, once individuals developed SCD, APOE ε4 conferred a 2.2x greater risk of developing some degree of objective cognitive impairment before death. Moreover, while non-converting "complainers" spent $M = 9.9$ years with

SCD before death, this time was reduced to $M = 5.9$ years in those with APOE ε4. It was not clear, however, whether this was due to a later onset of SCD among APOE ε4 carriers or earlier mortality due to neurocognitive pathology or other causes. Dubois et al. [55] elaborate on this interaction further. In their large sample of community-dwelling and medical help seeking individuals with SCD, APOE ε4-positive genotype increased the risk of conversion to AD only in the context of high amyloid burden. Specifically, the presence of APOE ε4 increased the risk of conversion to AD from 0.78% per year among non-carriers to 3.24% per year among carriers. The specific risk posed by APOE ε4 in the context of amyloid burden may help to explain the unequal risk of conversion posed by APOE ε4 across diagnostic groups (e.g., SCD, MCI, AD).

Discussion

The goals of this review were to a) determine whether APOE ε4 genotype occurred more frequently in individuals with SCD relative to other groups, b) to explore whether the occurrence of APOE ε4 in individuals with SCD increased their risk of later conversion to AD, and c) to present evidence of other sequelae or outcomes related to the co-occurrence of APOE ε4 genotype and SCD. Rather than merely consolidating and clarifying the data, the findings of this review highlight the complexity of the relationship between SCD, APOE ε4, and AD. As our knowledge of the mechanisms underlying pathological cognitive decline are yet inchoate, the mixed results of this review may not be entirely unexpected. Less expected may be that there were no clear systematic differences between studies using clinical or community samples, or those conducted cross-sectionally versus longitudinally, as might have been expected [44].

With regard to our initial objective, a univariate ANOVA was conducted to compare APOE ε4-positive prevalence across 25 studies that provided explicit frequency data. The frequency of APOE ε4 among healthy control groups in this review ($M = 24.48\%$) was comparable to APOE ε4 prevalence rates reported elsewhere in similar ethno-geographic groups [36,61,62], suggesting that the samples used in this review were likely ecologically representative. There was no significant difference in the prevalence of APOE ε4 between healthy controls and those with SCD ($M = 28.60\%$). In contrast, APOE ε4 frequency was significantly higher in cognitively impaired samples (i.e., MCI, diagnosed or probable AD) than those with SCD [63]. These results suggest that APOE ε4 may not be directly related to the development of SCD in healthy individuals, but that those predisposed to objective cognitive impairment are significantly more likely to carry an APOE ε4 allele. By extension, this may also suggest that those APOE ε4-carriers with SCD are more likely to decline than their non-carrier counterparts; however, without clear evidence of SCD prior to objective decline among MCI and AD samples, this conclusion is precarious at best.

The comparable APOE ε4 frequency between SCD and healthy control samples is consistent with previous evidence that SCD is more strongly related to older age [8], current or historical depression [8,64–66], anxiety [44,67], and/or other personality factors [66,68] than APOE ε4 status. Nevertheless, there may be reason to call the validity of this null effect into question. The increased frequency of APOE ε4 among those with MCI and AD relative to SCD and healthy controls may reflect systematic differences between clinical and community samples more than "true" differences in APOE ε4 frequency. In the current review, MCI and AD participants were far more likely to be sampled from memory clinics and university hospitals than were those with SCD or healthy controls. As such, these objectively impaired groups may disproportionately represent those with "pure" pathology (e.g., with few comorbid health concerns), as well as greater distress, education, and access to care. In addition, it is likely that there is substantially greater variability within SCD samples than other groups. Due to historically shifting criteria and terminology, the studies included in this review used a variety of operational definitions to identify SCD and SCD-equivalent groups. Moreover, the common categorization schemes used (e.g., asking whether individuals are concerned about their cognitive changes) tend to be poor at differentiating individuals with normative or anxious concerns from those with prodromal AD. Although Jessen et al.'s *SCD-Plus* guidelines [15] were explicitly developed for this purpose, few of the included studies used these criteria to define their SCD samples, not unexpected, given the recency of these criteria. Finally, unlike AD or even MCI, SCD does not imply a single underlying etiology, and in fact could be due to multiple etiologies. As such, it is possible that the consequent heterogeneity in SCD and SCD-equivalent samples may contribute to a dilution of significant differences in APOE status between SCD and healthy control samples.

This latter interpretation may be supported by pathophysiological evidence that, relative to healthy controls, those with SCD incur significantly greater risk of cognitive decline when APOE ε4 is present. Cross-sectional studies generally found that the presence of at least one APOE ε4 allele was associated with a greater degree of AD-consistent pathology in individuals with SCD, including increased amyloid deposition [52,56–58], possibly greater cortical atrophy [46,47,50], and potential white matter disruption [47]. However, it is difficult to know what such cross-sectional evidence may mean for a degenerative condition like SCD/prodromal AD. On the one hand, single time point designs remain vulnerable to the diluting effects of SCD group heterogeneity so any evidence of significant differences between healthy controls and SCD samples may be expected to be even greater than indicated. On the other hand, whether individuals with cognitive complaints are presenting with normative age-related behavior, exhibiting symptoms of depression and/or anxiety, or suffering from objective-impairment-heralding SCD may not become clear for a decade or more [41], calling the validity of these results into question. Thus, longitudinal evidence may be more convincing. There was general consensus between the longitudinal studies reviewed that SCD status and APOE ε4-positive genotype not only increase the risk of developing objective cognitive impairment as individual risk factors, but that they present exponentially greater risk when combined [8,56,59].

Taken together, the evidence garnered by the reviewed studies clearly identify APOE ε4 as a risk factor – with one important caveat: APOE ε4 may increase the risk of developing MCI, but may not confer any direct risk of developing AD. Brainerd and colleagues agree that APOE ε4 increases the risk of initial conversion from unimpaired to MCI; however, they argue that any apparent increases in AD risk are a redundancy due to a high proportion of MCI conversions per se [33]. This is echoed by others who argue that APOE ε4 status adds little predictive power above and beyond standardized testing once individuals are objectively impaired as, at that point, APOE ε4 status and impaired test performance explain overlapping variance [69,70]. Thus, it is clear that APOE ε4 is a strong predictor of cognitive decline in those with SCD, however, it may represent a more general risk of conversion to a cognitively impaired state than to AD per se; as AD remains the most common form of dementia, APOE ε4 may still pose a probabilistic risk of developing AD for those with SCD but may be better conceptualized as a general risk factor for MCI and its various outcomes. This finding is consistent with the rationale of Jack et al.'s decision to exclude APOE ε4 genotype as a diagnostic criterion in the most recent NIA-AA research framework for AD [22]. According to this framework, reliable AD diagnosis is argued to rely solely on biomarker profile. These biomarkers include Aβ and tau but, notably, exclude APOE ε4 genotype as it was neither necessary for the development of AD nor indicative of any specific stage of AD pathology [22].

It is important to note that, while the results of this review found APOE ε4 to be a robust risk biomarker for cognitive decline in those with SCD, APOE ε4-positive genotype is not deterministic and should not be expected to supplant other known dementia risk factors that confer orthogonal risk (such as vascular disease). For example, several studies have found that poor performance on standardized tests of memory are more predictive of conversion from SCD to MCI than the number of complaints or anxious/depressive symptomology, even when APOE ε4 was accounted for [71,72]. Others have found a constellation of objective memory decline, cognitive concern, and consistent SCD-related complaints over time to predict conversion to AD significantly better than APOE ε4 alone [73]. Aside from the additional sources of MCI/AD risk, protective factors are also likely to moderate the impact of APOE ε4 genetic risk. Education of at least eight years early in life has been found to be protective against later-life cognitive decline, with additional education being increasingly protective due to secondary outcomes (e.g., increased income) [72]. Related, educational achievement is known to correspond to cognitive reserve which itself has been found to delay the advent of objective cognitive symptoms in those with SCD, if not slow the pathological process once it is underway [74]. It is possible that, whatever pathology-hastening or -predisposing effect APOE ε4 may have is partially mitigated by these protective factors.

Clinical Implications

In light of this evidence, the insensitivity of standardized tests to the earliest potential signs of decline, and the currently ambiguous clinical picture presented by SCD, APOE ε4 testing may appear ripe for wide-scale adoption as a clinical screening tool. It is granted that APOE ε4 testing offers a non-invasive, low-cost, and effective complementary means [38] to identify complainants who may have prodromal AD [15]. However, given the mounting evidence linking AD with cardiovascular risk factors [75–78] and the significantly greater power of APOE ε4 to predict unspecific MCI than AD [33], APOE ε4 may be more likely to represent a general risk factor for pathological cognitive decline than genetic predisposition for AD specifically. Nevertheless, positive APOE ε4 screening may still serve to identify those most likely to benefit from lifestyle interventions (e.g., Mediterranean diet, aerobic exercise), as these methods have been shown to benefit individuals with MCI/dementia equally regardless of etiology [79–81].

Aside from diagnostic and treatment considerations, the non-specific nature of APOE ε4-related risk may introduce novel ethical considerations as well. For example, disseminating APOE ε4 status and its associated potential for risk may be particularly fraught as laypersons may be more inclined to perceive genotype as deterministic of future outcomes. If inadequately addressed, this fundamental misunderstanding is liable to cause a high degree of undue distress and, in extreme situations, may endanger individuals' current functioning. As such, employing genetic testing within a medical context may behoove a greater degree of clinical competency and/or specialized training [82]. A more novel consideration may be the impact of direct-to-consumer genetic testing on SCD. Given the recent proliferation of personal DNA testing kits, individuals with SCD may now readily access genetic information that is particularly prone to over-interpretation and misconstrual without the mitigating influence of medical insight. It is plausible that individuals with SCD may not only be more motivated to seek genetic testing to corroborate the veracity of their concerns, but that they may preferentially attend to information that reinforces their greatest fears. Conversely, at-home genetic testing may also influence the incidence of SCD. Although genetic testing is often pursued for medical purposes, a growing number of people may engage in genetic testing for more benign purposes, such as exploring ancestry and casual interest. In light of the growing public awareness of Alzheimer's disease and its various genetic risk factors, it is possible that incidental findings of APOE ε4-positive genotype may incline individuals otherwise unconcerned about their cognitive status toward hypervigilance for cognitive slips and increased anxiety in their event. As a comprehensive exploration of the full scope of ethical considerations and implications of genotype testing and disclosure is beyond the scope of the current review, the reader is directed to excellent articles by Schicktanz et al. [83], Green et al. [84], and Hawkins and Ho [85] for further discussion of these topics.

Future Directions

Several recommendations for future study emerged from this review. Firstly, there was heterogeneity in the terminology and classification schemes used across SCD studies. Although a number of the included studies were conducted before the establishment of the *SCD-Plus* criteria [15], many were not. While it is granted that the *SCD-Plus* criteria require further refinement, it is the most robust metric of SCD-conversion risk currently available. Continued use of idiosyncratic criteria and measures to classify SCD adds variance to our joint understanding of SCD risk, trajectory, and characteristic features. For this reason, it is recommended that future studies strongly consider adopting the *SCD-Plus* criteria as an ersatz "gold standard method" to classify their respective SCD samples. Secondly, though a more standardized categorization of SCD would lend more credence to cross-sectional findings, the longer-term and potentially degenerative nature of SCD implores further longitudinal investigation. At this time, few studies have been dedicated to exploring cognitive change, structural change, mood, or self-perceptions over the course of decline from SCD. A greater understanding of these longitudinal aspects may help establish a greater clinical recognition of SCD and a greater awareness of whether individuals are declining, what a typical degenerative trajectory may look like, and where in the trajectory they may fall. Thirdly, there has been considerable concern regarding potentially confounding effects of sample type (i.e., community vs. clinic). Although the current study did not find a significant effect of sample type on APOE ε4 frequency, AD samples may be uniquely difficult to access in the community. Given evidence that APOE ε4 may uniquely confer risk for conversion to MCI (and not AD directly), it is recommended that more work focus specifically on understanding this relationship. Doing so may not only preclude the need for AD samples and the potential interference of sample type but may also serve to focus the scope of current research efforts on the active link between APOE ε4, SCD, and cognitive decline. Finally, the majority of longitudinal evidence regarding the effects of SCD and APOE ε4 on AD conversion was derived from community-based samples. Although this arguably provides more representative data regarding the influence of SCD and APOE ε4 generally, given the potential application of this literature to clinical contexts, community-based studies may provide limited insight into the characteristics of those presenting to general or specialized clinics. Therefore, further longitudinal exploration of SCD-APOE ε4 interactions in medical help-seeking individuals (i.e., clinical samples) is merited.

Conclusion

In conclusion, this review found that APOE ε4 was no more likely to occur in the SCD or SCD-equivalent samples used versus healthy controls without cognitive concerns, but that APOE ε4 carriers were more likely to develop objective cognitive impairment. Specifically, having an APOE ε4 allele did not predispose individuals to develop SCD but it did confer additional risk of increased amyloid deposition, non-normative cortical atrophy, and eventual pathological cognitive decline in those who already reported cognitive concerns. As encouraging as these results may be, however, the exact role played by APOE ε4 in the development of AD or other objective cognitive impairment continues to be unclear due to a lack of convergent evidence and considerable sample heterogeneity. Consequently, further investigation is warranted before APOE ε4 genetic testing can be recommended for wide-scale clinical adoption as a viable diagnostic/screening tool for pathological cognitive decline.

Conflict of Interest/Disclosure Statement

JIA receives financial support from the Alzheimer Society of Canada: Alzheimer Society Research Program/Dr. and Mrs. Albert Spatz Award. The authors have no other disclosures or conflicts of interest to report.

References

[1]   He W, Goodkind D, Kowal P (2015) *An Aging World: 2015 International Population Reports*, U.S. Government Publishing Office, Washington, DC.

[2]   Hebert LE, Weuve J, Scherr PA, Evans DA (2013) Alzheimer disease in the United States (2010-2050) estimated using the 2010 census. *Neurology* **80**, 1778–1783.

[3]   Aiello Bowles EJ, Larson EB, Pong RP, Walker RL, Anderson ML, Yu O, Gray SL, Crane PK, Dublin S (2016) Anesthesia exposure and risk of dementia and Alzheimer's disease: A prospective study. *J. Am. Geriatr. Soc.* **64**, 602–607.

[4]   Ohara T, Ninomiya T, Hata J, Ozawa M, Yoshida D, Mukai N, Nagata M, Iwaki T, Kitazono T, Kanba S, Kiyohara Y (2015) Midlife and late-life smoking and risk of dementia in the community: The Hisayama study. *J. Am. Geriatr. Soc.* **63**, 2332–2339.

[5]   Studart Neto A, Nitrini R (2016) Subjective cognitive decline: The first clinical manifestation of Alzheimer's disease? *Dement. Neuropsychol.* **10**, 170–177.

[6]   Jessen F (2014) Subjective and objective cognitive decline at the pre-dementia stage of Alzheimer's disease. *Eur. Arch. Psychiatry Clin. Neurosci.* **264 Suppl**, S3–7.

[7]   Reisberg B, Shulman MB, Torossian C, Leng L, Zhu W (2010) Outcome over seven years of healthy adults with and without subjective cognitive impairment. *Neuropsychol. Rev.* **6**, 11–24.

[8]   Dik MG, Jonker C, Comijs HC, Bouter LM, Twisk JW, van Kamp GJ, Deeg DJ (2001) Memory complaints and APOE-epsilon4 accelerate cognitive decline in cognitively normal elderly. *Neurology* **57**, 2217–2222.

[9]   van Harten AC, Visser PJ, Pijnenburg YAL, Teunissen CE, Blankenstein MA, Scheltens P, van der Flier WM (2017) Cerebrospinal fluid AB42 is the best predictor of clinical progression in patients with subjective complaints. 1–7.

[10] Perrotin A, Mormino EC, Madison CM, Hayenga AO, Jagust WJ (2012) Subjective cognition and amyloid deposition imaging: A Pittsburgh compound B positron emission tomography study in normal elderly individuals. *Arch. Neurol.* **69**, 223–229.

[11] Visser PJ, Verhey F, Knol DL, Scheltens P, Wahlund L-O, Freund-Levi Y, Tsolaki M, Minthon L, Wallin ÅK, Hampel H, Bürger K, Pirttila T, Soininen H, Rikkert MO, Verbeek MM, Spiru L, Blennow K (2009) Prevalence and prognostic value of CSF markers of Alzheimer's disease pathology in patients with subjective cognitive impairment or mild cognitive impairment in the DESCRIPA study: A prospective cohort study. *Lancet Neurol.* **8**, 619–627.

[12] Simmons BB, Hartmann B, Dejoseph D (2011) Evaluation of suspected dementia. *Ratio*.

[13] Hong JY, Sunwoo MK, Chung SJ, Ham JH, Lee JE, Sohn YH, Lee PH (2014) Subjective cognitive decline predicts future deterioration in cognitively normal patients with Parkinson's disease. *Neurobiol. Aging* **35**, 1739–1743.

[14] Slot RER, Van Harten AC, Kester MI, Jongbloed W, Bouwman FH, Teunissen CE, Scheltens P, Veerhuis R, Van Der Flier WM (2017) Apolipoprotein A1 in cerebrospinal fluid and plasma and progression to Alzheimer's disease in non-demented elderly. *J. Alzheimer's Dis.* **56**, 687–697.

[15] Jessen F, Amariglio RE, van Boxtel M, Breteler M, Ceccaldi M, Chételat G, Dubois B, Dufouil C, Ellis KA, van der Flier WM, Glodzik L, van Harten AC, de Leon MJ, McHugh P, Mielke MM, Molinuevo JL, Mosconi L, Osorio RS, Perrotin A, Petersen RC, Rabin LA, Rami L, Reisberg B, Rentz DM, Sachdev PS, de la Sayette V, Saykin AJ, Scheltens P, Shulman MB, Slavin MJ, Sperling RA, Stewart R, Uspenskaya O, Vellas B, Visser PJ, Wagner M, Subjective Cognitive Decline Initiative (SCD-I) Working Group (2014) A conceptual framework for research on subjective cognitive decline in preclinical

Alzheimer's disease. *Neuropsychol. Rev.* **10**, 844–852.

[16]   Molinuevo JL, Rabin LA, Amariglio R, Buckley R, Dubois B, Ellis KA, Ewers M, Hampel H, Klöppel S, Rami L, Reisberg B, Saykin AJ, Sikkes S, Smart CM, Snitz BE, Sperling R, van der Flier WM, Wagner M, Jessen F, Group SCDIS-IW (2017) Implementation of subjective cognitive decline criteria in research studies. *Alzheimer's Dement.* 1–16.

[17]   Fonseca JAS, Ducksbury R, Rodda J, Whitfield T, Nagaraj C, Suresh K, Stevens T, Walker Z (2015) Factors that predict cognitive decline in patients with subjective cognitive impairment. *Int. Psychogeriatr.* **27**, 1671–1677.

[18]   Rabin LA, Smart CM, Crane PK, Amariglio RE, Berman LM, Boada M, Buckley RF, Chételat G, Dubois B, Ellis KA, Gifford KA, Jefferson AL, Jessen F, Katz MJ, Lipton RB, Luck T, Maruff P, Mielke MM, Molinuevo JL, Naeem F, Perrotin A, Petersen RC, Rami L, Reisberg B, Rentz DM, Riedel-Heller SG, Risacher SL, Rodriguez O, Sachdev PS, Saykin AJ, Slavin MJ, Snitz BE, Sperling RA, Tandetnik C, van der Flier WM, Wagner M, Wolfsgruber S, Sikkes SAM (2015) Subjective cognitive decline in older adults: An overview of self-report measures used across 19 international research studies. *J. Alzheimers. Dis.* **48 Suppl 1**, S63–86.

[19]   Mulligan BP, Smart CM, Ali JI (2016) Relationship of subjective and objective performance indicators in subjective cognitive decline. *Psychol. Neurosci.* **9**, 362–378.

[20]   Rabin LA, Smart CM, Amariglio RE (2017) Subjective cognitive decline in preclinical Alzheimer's disease. *Annu. Rev. Clin. Psychol.* **13**, 369–396.

[21]   van Oijen, M., de Jong, F. J., Hofman, A., Koudstaal, P. J., & Breteler MMB (2007) Subjective memory complaints, education, and risk of Alzheimer's disease. *Alzheimer's Dement.* **3**, 92–97.

[22]   Jack CR, Bennett DA, Blennow K, Carrillo MC, Dunn B, Haeberlein SB, Holtzman DM, Jagust W, Jessen F, Karlawish J, Liu E, Molinuevo JL, Montine T, Phelps C, Rankin KP, Rowe CC, Scheltens P, Siemers E, Snyder HM, Sperling R, Elliott C, Masliah E, Ryan L, Silverberg N (2018) NIA-AA Research Framework: Toward a biological definition of Alzheimer's disease. *Alzheimer's Dement.* **14**, 535–562.

[23]   Allan CL, Ebmeier KP (2011) The influence of ApoE4 on clinical progression of dementia: A meta-analysis. *Int. J. Geriatr. Psychiatry* **26**, 520–526.

[24]   Chen K-L, Sun Y-M, Zhou Y, Zhao Q-H, Ding D, Guo Q-H (2016) Associations between APOE polymorphisms and seven diseases with cognitive impairment including Alzheimer's disease, frontotemporal dementia, and dementia with Lewy bodies in southeast China. *Psychiatr. Genet.* **26**, 124–131.

[25]   Jiang S, Tang L, Zhao N, Yang W, Qiu Y, Chen H-Z (2016) A systems view of the differences between APOE ε4 carriers and non-carriers in Alzheimer's disease. *Front. Aging Neurosci.* **8**, 2990.

[26]   Liu Y, Tan L, Wang H-F, Liu Y, Hao X-K, Tan C-C, Jiang T, Liu B, Zhang D-Q, Yu J-T, Alzheimer's Disease Neuroimaging Initiative (2016) Multiple effect of APOE genotype on clinical and neuroimaging biomarkers across Alzheimer's disease spectrum. *Mol. Neurobiol.* **53**, 4539–4547.

[27]   Mata IF, Leverenz JB, Weintraub D, Trojanowski JQ, Hurtig HI, Van Deerlin VM, Ritz B, Rausch R, Rhodes SL, Factor SA, Wood-Siverio C, Quinn JF, Chung KA, Peterson AL, Espay AJ, Revilla FJ, Devoto J, Hu S-C, Cholerton BA, Wan JY, Montine TJ, Edwards KL, Zabetian CP (2014) APOE, MAPT, and SNCA genes and cognitive performance in Parkinson disease. *JAMA Neurol.* **71**, 1405–1412.

[28]   Pink A, Stokin GB, Bartley MM, Roberts RO, Sochor O, Machulda MM, Krell-Roesch J,

Knopman DS, Acosta JI, Christianson TJ, Pankratz VS, Mielke MM, Petersen RC, Geda YE (2015) Neuropsychiatric symptoms, APOE ε4, and the risk of incident dementia: A population-based study. *Neurology* **84**, 935–943.

[29]   Prestia A, Caroli A, Wade SK, van der Flier WM, Ossenkoppele R, Van Berckel B, Barkhof F, Teunissen CE, Wall A, Carter SF, Schöll M, Choo IH, Nordberg A, Scheltens P, Frisoni GB (2015) Prediction of AD dementia by biomarkers following the NIA-AA and IWG diagnostic criteria in MCI patients from three European memory clinics. *Neuropsychol. Rev.* **11**, 1191–1201.

[30]   Puglielli, L., Tanzi, R. E., Kovacs DM (2003) Alzheimer's disease: The cholesterol connection. *Nat. Neurosci.* **6**, 345–351.

[31]   Ward A, Crean S, Mercaldi CJ, Collins JM, Boyd D, Cook MN, Arrighi HM (2012) Prevalence of apolipoprotein E4 genotype and homozygotes (APOE e4/4) among patients diagnosed with Alzheimer's disease: A systematic review and meta-analysis. *Neuroepidemiology* **38**, 1–17.

[32]   Scarabino D, Broggio E, Gambina G, Maida C, Gaudio MR, Corbo RM (2016) Apolipoprotein E genotypes and plasma levels in mild cognitive impairment conversion to Alzheimer's disease: A follow-up study. *Am. J. Med. Genet. B. Neuropsychiatr. Genet.* **171**, 1131–1138.

[33]   Brainerd CJ, Reyna VF, Petersen RC, Smith GE, Kenney AE, Gross CJ, Taub ES, Plassman BL, Fisher GG (2013) The apolipoprotein E genotype predicts longitudinal transitions to mild cognitive impairment but not to Alzheimer's dementia: Findings from a nationally representative study. *Neuropsychology* **27**, 86–94.

[34]   Farrer LA, Cupples AL, Kukull WA, Mayeux R, Myers RH, Pericak-Vance MA, Farrer LA, Cupples LA, Haines JL, Hyman B, Kukull WA, Mayeux R, Myers RH, Pericak-

Vance MA, Risch N, van Duijn CM (1997) Effects of age, sex, and ethnicity on the association between apolipoprotein E genotype and Alzheimer disease. *JAMA J. Am. Med. Assoc.* **278**, 1349–1356.

[35] Tschanz JT, Welsh-Bohmer KA, Lyketsos CG, Corcoran C, Green RC, Hayden K, Norton MC, Zandi PP, Toone L, West NA, Breitner JCS, Cache County Investigators (2006) Conversion to dementia from mild cognitive disorder: The Cache County Study. *Neurology* **67**, 229–234.

[36] Alzgene - meta-analysis of all published AD association studies (case-control only) APOE_E2/3/4, Last updated 2010, Accessed on 2010.

[37] Edmonds EC, Delano-Wood L, Galasko DR, Salmon DP, Bondi MW (2016) Subtle cognitive decline and biomarker staging in preclinical Alzheimer's disease. *J. Alzheimer's Dis.* **47**, 231–242.

[38] Yi L, Wu T, Luo W, Zhou W, Wu J (2014) A non-invasive, rapid method to genotype late-onset Alzheimer's disease-related apolipoprotein E gene polymorphisms. *Neural Regen. Res.* **9**, 69–75.

[39] Canadian Psychological Association (2000) *Canadian code of ethics for psychologists - third edition*, Canadian Psychological Association, Ottawa, ON.

[40] Smart CM, Karr JE, Areshenkoff CN, Rabin LA, Hudon C, Gates N, Ali JI, Arenaza-Urquijo EM, Buckley RF, Chételat G, Hampel H, Jessen F, Marchant NL, Sikkes SAM, Tales A, van der Flier WM, Wesselman L (2017) Non-pharmacologic interventions for older adults with subjective cognitive decline: Systematic review, meta-analysis, and preliminary recommendations. *Neuropsychol. Rev.* **27**, 245–257.

[41] Reisberg B, Gauthier S (2008) Current evidence for subjective cognitive impairment (SCI) as the pre-mild cognitive impairment (MCI) stage of subsequently manifest Alzheimer's

disease. *Int. Psychogeriatr.* **20**, 1–16.

[42]   Liu C-C, Liu C-C, Kanekiyo T, Xu H, Bu G (2013) Apolipoprotein E and Alzheimer
       disease: risk, mechanisms and therapy. *Nat. Rev. Neurol.* **9**, 106–118.

[43]   Small GW, Chen ST, Komo S, Ercoli L, Bookheimer S, Miller K, Lavretsky H, Saxena S,
       Kaplan A, Dorsey D, Scott WK, Saunders AM, Haines JL, Roses AD, Pericak-Vance MA
       (1999) Memory self-appraisal in middle-aged and older adults with the apolipoprotein E-4
       allele. *Am. J. Psychiatry* **156**, 1035–1038.

[44]   Perrotin A, La Joie R, de la Sayette V, Barré L, Mézenge F, Mutlu J, Guilloteau D, Egret
       S, Eustache F, Chételat G (2017) Subjective cognitive decline in cognitively normal elders
       from the community or from a memory clinic: Differential affective and imaging
       correlates. *Neuropsychol. Rev.* **13**, 550–560.

[45]   Cohen J, Cohen P (2002) *Applied multiple regression/correlation analysis for the
       behavioral sciences, 3rd Ed.*, Routledge, Hillsdale, NJ.

[46]   Striepens N, Scheef L, Wind A, Meiberth D, Popp J, Spottke A, Kölsch H, Wagner M,
       Jessen F (2011) Interaction effects of subjective memory impairment and ApoE4 genotype
       on episodic memory and hippocampal volume. *Psychol. Med.* **41**, 1997–2006.

[47]   Lee Y-M, Ha J-K, Park J-M, Lee B-D, Moon E, Chung Y-I, Kim J-H, Kim H-J, Mun C-
       W, Kim T-H, Kim Y-H (2015) Impact of apolipoprotein E4 polymorphism on the gray
       matter volume and the white matter integrity in subjective memory impairment without
       white matter hyperintensities: Voxel-based morphometry and tract-based spatial statistics
       study under 3-Tesla MRI. *J. Neuroimaging* **26**, 144–149.

[48]   Bartley M, Bokde AL, Ewers M, Faluyi YO, Tobin WO, Snow A, Connolly J, Delaney C,
       Coughlan T, Collins DR, Hampel H, O'Neill D (2011) Subjective memory complaints in
       community dwelling healthy older people: The influence of brain and psychopathology.

Int. J. Geriatr. Psychiatry **27**, 836–843.

[49]   Watfa G, Marteau JB, Rossignol P, Kearney-Schwartz A, Fay R, Bracard S, Felblinger J, Boivin JM, Lacolley P, Visvikis-Siest S, Benetos A, Zannad F (2010) Association study of gene polymorphisms involved in vascular alterations in elderly hypertensives with subjective memory complaints. *Dement. Geriatr. Cogn. Disord.* **30**, 440–448.

[50]   Stewart R, Godin O, Crivello F, Maillard P, Mazoyer B, Tzourio C, Dufouil C (2011) Longitudinal neuroimaging correlates of subjective memory impairment: 4-year prospective community study. *Br. J. Psychiatry* **198**, 199–205.

[51]   Cherbuin N, Sargent-Cox K, Easteal S, Sachdev P, Anstey KJ (2015) Hippocampal atrophy is associated with subjective memory decline: The PATH through life study. *Am. J. Geriatr. Psychiatry* **23**, 546–556.

[52]   Risacher SL, Kim S, Nho K, Foroud T, Shen L, Petersen RC, Jack CR, Beckett LA, Aisen PS, Koeppe RA, Jagust WJ, Shaw LM, Trojanowski JQ, Weiner MW, Saykin AJ, Alzheimer's Disease Neuroimaging Initiative (ADNI) (2015) APOE effect on Alzheimer's disease biomarkers in older adults with significant memory concern. *Alzheimer's Dement.* **11**, 1417–1429.

[53]   Chételat G, Villemagne VL, Pike KE, Baron JC, Bourgeat P, Jones G, Faux NG, Ellis KA, Salvado O, Szoeke C, Martins RN, Ames D, Masters CL, Rowe CC (2010) Larger temporal volume in elderly with high versus low beta-amyloid deposition. *Brain* **133**, 3349–3358.

[54]   Mattsson N, Insel PS, Donohue M, Landau S, Jagust WJ, Shaw LM, Trojanowski JQ, Zetterberg H, Blennow K, Weiner MW (2014) Independent information from cerebrospinal fluid amyloid-β and florbetapir imaging in Alzheimer's disease. *Brain* **138**, 772–783.

[55]   Dubois B, Epelbaum S, Nyasse F, Bakardjian H, Gagliardi G, Uspenskaya O, Houot M,

Lista S, Cacciamani F, Potier MC, Bertrand A, Lamari F, Benali H, Mangin JF, Colliot O,

Genthon R, Habert MO, Hampel H, Audrain C, Auffret A, Baldacci F, Benakki I, Bertin

H, Boukadida L, Cavedo E, Chiesa P, Dauphinot L, Dos Santos A, Dubois M, Durrleman

S, Fontaine G, Genin A, Glasman P, Jungalee N, Kas A, Kilani M, La Corte V, Lehericy

S, Letondor C, Levy M, Lowrey M, Ly J, Makiese O, Metzinger C, Michon A, Mochel F,

Poisson C, Ratovohery S, Revillon M, Rojkova K, Roy P, Santos-Andrade K, Schindler R,

Seux L, Simon V, Sole M, Tandetnik C, Teichmann M, Thiebaut de Shotten M, Younsi N

(2018) Cognitive and neuroimaging features and brain β-amyloidosis in individuals at risk

of Alzheimer's disease (INSIGHT-preAD): a longitudinal observational study. *Lancet*

Neurol. **17**, 335–346.

[56]   Kryscio RJ, Abner EL, Cooper GE, Fardo DW, Jicha GA, Nelson PT, Smith CD, Van

Eldik LJ, Schmitt LWFA (2014) Self-reported memory complaints: Implications from a

longitudinal cohort with autopsies. *Neurology* **83**, 1359–1365.

[57]   Zwan MD, Villemagne VL, Doré V, Buckley R, Bourgeat P, Veljanoski R, Salvado O,

Williams R, Margison L, Rembach A, Macaulay SL, Martins R, Ames D, van der Flier

WM, Ellis KA, Scheltens P, Masters CL, Rowe CC (2016) Subjective memory complaints

in APOE e4 carriers are associated with high amyloid-β burden. *J. Alzheimer's Dis.* **49**,

1115–1122.

[58]   Rowe CC, Ellis KA, Rimajova M, Bourgeat P, Pike KE, Jones G, Fripp J, Tochon-Danguy

H, Morandeau L, O'Keefe G, Price R, Raniga P, Robins P, Acosta O, Lenzo N, Szoeke C,

Salvado O, Head R, Martins R, Masters CL, Ames D, Villemagne VL (2010) Amyloid

imaging results from the Australian Imaging, Biomarkers and Lifestyle (AIBL) study of

aging. *Neurobiol. Aging* **31**, 1275–1283.

[59]   Hong YJ, Yoon B, Shim YS, Kim S-O, Kim HJ, Choi SH, Jeong JH, Yoon SJ, Yang DW, Lee J-H (2015) Predictors of clinical progression of subjective memory impairment in elderly subjects: Data from the Clinical Research Centers for Dementia of South Korea (CREDOS). *Dement. Geriatr. Cogn. Disord.* **40**, 158–165.

[60]   Jessen F, Wolfsgruber S, Wiese B, Bickel H, M??sch E, Kaduszkiewicz H, Pentzek M, Riedel-Heller SG, Luck T, Fuchs A, Weyerer S, Werle J, Van Den Bussche H, Scherer M, Maier W, Wagner M (2014) AD dementia risk in late MCI, in early MCI, and in subjective memory impairment. *Alzheimer's Dement.* **10**, 76–83.

[61]   Corbo RM, Scacchi R (1999) Apolipoprotein E (APOE) allele distribution in the world. Is APOE*4 a "thrift" allele? . *Ann. Hum. Genet.* **63**, 301–310.

[62]   Ghebranious N, Ivacic L, Mallum J, Dokken C (2005) Detection of ApoE E2, E3 and E4 alleles using MALDI-TOF mass spectrometry and the homogeneous mass-extend technology. *Nucleic Acids Res.* **33**, 1–6.

[63]   Verdile G, Laws SM, Henley D, Ames D, Bush AI, Ellis KA, Faux NG, Gupta VB, Li Q-X, Masters CL, Pike KE, Rowe CC, Szoeke C, Taddei K, Villemagne VL, Martins RN (2012) Associations between gonadotropins, testosterone and β amyloid in men at risk of Alzheimer's disease. *Mol. Psychiatry* **19**, 69–75.

[64]   Jessen F, Wiese B, Cvetanovska G, Fuchs A, Kaduszkiewicz H, Kölsch H, Luck T, Mösch E, Pentzek M, Riedel-Heller SG, Werle J, Weyerer S, Zimmerman T, Maier W, Bickel H (2007) Patterns of subjective memory impairment in the elderly: Association with memory performance. *Psychol. Med.* **37**, 1753–1762.

[65]   Stewart R, Russ C, Richards M, Brayne C, Lovestone S, Mann A (2001) Depression, APOE genotype and subjective memory impairment: A cross-sectional study in an African-Caribbean population. *Psychol. Med.* **31**, 431–440.

[66]   Studer J, Donati A, Popp J, von Gunten A (2014) Subjective cognitive decline in patients
       with mild cognitive impairment and healthy older adults: Association with personality
       traits. *Geriatr. Gerontol. Int.* **14**, 589–595.

[67]   Tandetnik C, Hergueta T, Bonnet P, Dubois B, Bungener C (2017) Influence of early
       maladaptive schemas, depression, and anxiety on the intensity of self-reported cognitive
       complaint in older adults with subjective cognitive decline. *Int. Psychogeriatr.* **90**, 1–11.

[68]   Snitz BE, Lopez OL, McDade E, Becker JT, Cohen AD, Price JC, Mathis CA, Klunk WE
       (2015) Amyloid-β imaging in older adults presenting to a memory clinic with subjective
       cognitive decline: A pilot study. *J. Alzheimer's Dis.* **48**, S151–S159.

[69]   Fleisher AS, Sowell BB, Taylor C, Gamst AC, Petersen RC, Thal LJ (2007) Clinical
       predictors of progression to Alzheimer disease in amnestic mild cognitive impairment.
       Neurology **68**, 1588–1595..

[70]   Luis CA, Barker WW, Loewenstein DA, Crum TA, Rogaeva E, Kawarai T, St. George-
       Hyslop P, Duara R (2004) Conversion to dementia among two groups with cognitive
       impairment: A preliminary report. *Dement. Geriatr. Cogn. Disord.* **18**, 307–313.

[71]   Fernández-Blázquez MA, Ávila-Villanueva M, Maestú F, Medina M (2016) Specific
       features of subjective cognitive decline predict faster conversion to mild cognitive
       impairment. *J. Alzheimer's Dis.* **52**, 271–281.

[72]   Zahodne LB, Manly JJ, MacKay-Brandt A, Stern Y (2013) Cognitive declines precede and
       predict functional declines in aging and Alzheimer's disease. *PLoS One* **8**, e73645.

[73]   Wolfsgruber S, Kleineidam L, Wagner M, Mösch E, Bickel H, Lühmann D, Ernst A,
       Wiese B, Steinmann S, König HH, Brettschneider C, Luck T, Stein J, Weyerer S, Werle J,
       Pentzek M, Fuchs A, Maier W, Scherer M, Riedel-Heller SG, Jessen F (2016) Differential
       risk of incident Alzheimer's disease dementia in stable versus unstable patterns of

subjective cognitive decline. *J. Alzheimer's Dis.* **54**, 1135–1146.

[74]   Soldan A, Pettigrew C, Cai Q, Wang J, Wang MC, Moghekar A, Miller MI, Albert M (2017) Cognitive reserve and long-term change in cognition in aging and preclinical Alzheimer's disease. *Neurobiol. Aging* **60**, 164–172.

[75]   Beeri MS, Rapp M, Silverman JM, Schmeidler J, Grossman HT, Fallon JT, Purohit DP, Perl DP, Siddiqui A, Lesser G, Rosendorff C, Haroutunian V (2006) Coronary artery disease is associated with Alzheimer disease neuropathology in APOE4 carriers. *Neurology* **66**, 1399–1404.

[76]   Knopman DS, Gottesman RF, Sharrett AR, Wruck LM, Windham BG, Coker L, Schneider AL, Hengrui S, Alonso A, Coresh J, Albert MS, Mosley TH (2016) Mild cognitive impairment and dementia prevalence: The Atherosclerosis Risk in Communities Neurocognitive Study (ARIC-NCS). *Alzheimer's Dement. (Amsterdam, Netherlands)* **2**, 1–11.

[77]   Mielke M, Leoutsakos J, Tschanz J, Green R, Tripodis Y, Corcoran C, Norton M (2011) Interaction between vascular factors and the APOE E4 allele predict rate of progression in Alzheimer's dementia. *Alzheimer's Dement.* **7**, S598.

[78]   Snyder HM, Corriveau RA, Craft S, Faber JE, Greenberg SM, Knopman D, Lamb BT, Montine TJ, Nedergaard M, Schaffer CB, Schneider JA, Wellington C, Wilcock DM, Zipfel GJ, Zlokovic B, Bain LJ, Bosetti F, Galis ZS, Koroshetz W, Carrillo MC (2015) Vascular contributions to cognitive impairment and dementia including Alzheimer's disease. *Alzheimer's Dement.* **11**, 710–717.

[79]   Hernandez SS, Sandreschi PF, Silva FC, Arancibia BA, da Silva R, Gutierres PJ, Andrade A (2014) What are the benefits of exercise for Alzheimer's disease? A systematic review of past 10 years. *J Aging Phys Act* 659–668.

[80]   Morris JK, Vidoni ED, Johnson DK, Van Sciver A, Mahnken JD, Honea RA, Wilkins HM, Brooks WM, Billinger SA, Swerdlow RH, Burns JM (2017) Aerobic exercise for Alzheimer's disease: A randomized controlled pilot trial. *PLoS One* **12**, 1–14.

[81]   Tuokko, H. A., Smart CM (2018) *Neuropsychology of cognitive decline: A developmental approach to assessment and intervention*, Guilford Press, New York, NY.

[82]   Arribas-Ayllon M (2011) The ethics of disclosing genetic diagnosis for Alzheimer's disease: Do we need a new paradigm? *Br. Med. Bull.* **100**, 7–21.

[83]   Schicktanz S, Schweda M, Ballenger JF, Fox PJ, Halpern J, Kramer JH, Micco G, Post SG, Thompson C, Knight RT, Jagust WJ (2014) Before it is too late: Professional responsibilities in late-onset Alzheimer's research and pre-symptomatic prediction. *Front. Hum. Neurosci.* **8**.

[84]   Green RC, Christensen KD, Cupples LA, Relkin NR, Whitehouse PJ, Royal CDM, Obisesan TO, Cook-Deegan R, Linnenbringer E, Butson MB, Fasaye G-A, Levinson E, Roberts JS, REVEAL Study Group (2015) A randomized noninferiority trial of condensed protocols for genetic risk disclosure of Alzheimer's disease. *Neuropsychol. Rev.* **11**, 1222–1230.

[85]   Hawkins AK, Ho A (2012) Genetic counseling and the ethical issues around direct to consumer genetic testing. *J. Genet. Couns.* **21**, 367–373.

[86]   Jorm AF, Butterworth P, Anstey KJ, Christensen H, Easteal S, Maller J, Mather KA, Turakulov RI, Wen W, Sachdev P (2004) Memory complaints in a community sample aged 60-64 years: Associations with cognitive functioning, psychiatric symptoms, medical conditions, APOE genotype, hippocampus and amygdala volumes, and white-matter hyperintensities. *Psychol. Med.* **34**, 1495–506.

[87]   Maruyama M, Matsui T, Tanji H, Nemoto M, Tomita N, Ootsuki M, Arai H, Sasaki H

(2004) Cerebrospinal fluid tau protein and periventricular white matter lesions in patients with mild cognitive impairment. *Arch. Neurol.* **61**, 716.

[88] Lautenschlager NT, Wu JS, Laws SM, Almeida OP, Clarnette RM, Joesbury K, Wagenpfeil S, Martins G, Paton A, Gandy SE, Forstl H, Martins RN (2005) Neurological soft signs are associated with APOE genotype, age and cognitive performance. *J. Alzheimers Dis.* **7**, 325–330.

[89] Striepens N, Scheef L, Wind A, Popp J, Spottke A, Cooper-Mahkorn D, Suliman H, Wagner M, Schild HH, Jessen F (2010) Volume loss of the medial temporal lobe structures in subjective memory impairment. *Dement. Geriatr. Cogn. Disord.* **29**, 75–81.

[90] Fortea J, Sala-Llonch R, Bartrés-Faz D, Lladó A, Solé-Padullés C, Bosch B, Antonell A, Olives J, Sanchez-Valle R, Molinuevo JL, Rami L (2011) Cognitively preserved subjects with transitional cerebrospinal fluid β-amyloid 1-42 values have thicker cortex in Alzheimer's disease vulnerable areas. *Biol. Psychiatry* **70**, 183–190.

[91] Norberg J, Graff C, Almkvist O, Ewers M, Frisoni GB, Frölich L, Hampel H, Jones RW, Kehoe PG, Lenoir H, Minthon L, Nobili F, Olde Rikkert M, Rigaud AS, Scheltens P, Soininen H, Spiru L, Tsolaki M, Wahlund LO, Vellas B, Wilcock G, Elias-Sonnenschein LS, Verhey FRJ, Visser PJ (2011) Regional differences in effects of APOE ε4 on cognitive impairment in non-demented subjects. *Dement. Geriatr. Cogn. Disord.* **32**, 135–142.

[92] Smith CD, Andersen AH, Gold BT (2012) Structural brain alterations before mild cognitive impairment in ADNI: Validation of volume loss in a predefined antero-temporal region. *J. Alzheimer's Dis.* **31**, 49–58.

[93] Peavy GM, Santiago DP, Edland SD (2013) Subjective memory complaints are associated with diurnal measures of salivary cortisol in cognitively intact older adults. *Am. J. Geriatr.*

Psychiatry **21**, 925–928.

[94]   Hall A, Mattila J, Koikkalainen J, Lötjonen J, Wolz R, Scheltens P, Frisoni G, Tsolaki M, Nobili F, Freund-levi Y, Minthon L, Frölich L, Hampel H, Visser PJ, Soininen H (2015) Predicting progression from cognitive impairment to Alzheimer's disease with the Disease State Index. *Curr. Alzheimer Res.* **12**, 69–79.

[95]   Krell-Roesch J, Woodruff BK, Acosta JI, Locke DE, Hentz JG, Stonnington CM, Stokin GB, Nagle C, Michel BF, Sambuchi N, Caselli RJ, Geda YE (2015) APOE ε4 genotype and the risk for subjective cognitive impairment in elderly persons. *J. Neuropsychiatry Clin. Neurosci.* **27**, 322–325.

[96]   Dhilla Albers A, Asafu-Adjei J, Delaney MK, Kelly KE, Gomez-Isla T, Blacker D, Johnson KA, Sperling RA, Hyman BT, Betensky RA, Hastings L, Albers MW (2016) Episodic memory of odors stratifies Alzheimer biomarkers in normal elderly. *Ann. Neurol.* **80**, 846–857.

[97]   Sierra-Rio A, Balasa M, Olives J, Antonell A, Iranzo A, Castellví M, Bosch B, Grau-Rivera O, Fernandez-Villullas G, Rami L, Lladó A, Sánchez-Valle R, Molinuevo JL (2016) Cerebrospinal fluid biomarkers predict clinical evolution in patients with subjective cognitive decline and mild cognitive impairment. *Neurodegener. Dis.* **16**, 69–76.

[98]   Voevodskaya O, Sundgren PC, Strandberg O, Zetterberg H, Minthon L, Blennow K, Wahlund LO, Westman E, Hansson O (2016) Myo-inositol changes precede amyloid pathology and relate to APOE genotype in Alzheimer disease. *Neurology* **86**, 1754–1761.

[99]   Bridel C, Hoffmann T, Meyer A, Durieux S, Koel-Simmelink MA, Orth M, Scheltens P, Lues I, Teunissen CE (2017) Glutaminyl cyclase activity correlates with levels of Aβ peptides and mediators of angiogenesis in cerebrospinal fluid of Alzheimer's disease

patients. *Alzheimer's Res. Ther.* **9**, 1–11.

[100] Pařízková M, Andel R, Lerch O, Marková H, Gažová I, Vyhnálek M, Hort J, Laczó J
(2016) Homocysteine and real-space navigation performance among non-demented older
adults. *J. Alzheimer's Dis.* **55**, 951–964.

[101] Wirth M, Bejanin A, La Joie R, Arenaza-Urquijo EM, Gonneaud J, Landeau B, Perrotin A,
Mézenge F, de La Sayette V, Desgranges B, Chételat G (2018) Regional patterns of gray
matter volume, hypometabolism, and beta-amyloid in groups at risk of Alzheimer's
disease. *Neurobiol. Aging* **63**, 140–151.

Tables

Table 1.1: Summary of included studies (in order of publication date)

Study	SCD-Equivalent Classification	SCD n	SCD Mean Age (SD)	SCD % APOE-ε4	Sample Type
Dik et al., 2001 [8]	Memory complaints	298	72.8 (6.7)	26.8%	Community
Stewart et al., 2001[65]	Subjective memory impairment (SMI)	56	Range: 55-75[a]	32.0%[a]	Clinic
Maruyama et al., 2004 [87]	Memory complaints	15[b]	71.9 (4.1)[b]	10.7%[b]	Clinic
Lautenschlager et al., 2005 [88]	Subjective memory complaints (SMC)	121	74.7 (4.3)	19.8%	Community
Jessen et al., 2007 [64]	Subjective memory impairment (SMI)	1,093	80.1 (3.5)	20.3%	Community
Chételat et al., 2010 [53]	Subjective cognitive impairment (SCI)	49[a]	74.4 (6.8)[b]	26.5%[b]	Community
Rowe et al., 2010 [58]	Subjective memory complaints (SMC)	96	71.2 (7.4)	38.0%	Community
Striepens et al., 2010 [89]	Subjective memory impairment (SMI)	21	66.3 (6.2)	31.3%	Clinic
Watfa et al., 2010 [49]	Subjective memory complaints (SMC)	369	70.0 (6.0)	Undisclosed	Mixed
Bartley et al., 2011 [48]	Subjective memory complaints (SMC) - *Worriers* - *Non-worriers*	52 *31* *21*	Range: 55-85[c]	28.9	Community
Fortea at al., 2011 [90]	Subjective memory complaints (SMC)	16	69.7 (7.1)	20.0%	Clinic

[a] Data for total sample where SCD-specific data was not available
[b] Data for SCD at follow up only (regardless of baseline status or n)
[c] Data for total pooled SCD sample
[d] Data represents a purposefully matched sample of APOE+ to APOE-

Table 1 Continued

Study	SCD-Equivalent Classification	SCD n	SCD Mean Age (SD)	SCD % APOE-ε4	Sample Type
Norberg et al., 2011 [91]	Subjective cognitive impairment (SCI)	130	67.1 (7.4)	36.9%	Clinic
Stewart et al., 2011 [50]	Subjective memory impairment (SMI)	347	72.0 (4.0)[b]	21.9%[b]	Community
Striepens et al., 2011 [46]	Subjective memory impairment (SMI)	40	67.2 (6.6)	27.5%	Clinic
Smith et al., 2012 [92]	Memory complaints - *Converters* - *Non-converters*	53 *16* *37*	76.2 (4.4) *76.7 (5.1)* *75.9 (4.1)*	26.0% *44.0%* *19.0%*	Clinic
Verdile et al., 2012 [63]	Subjective memory complaints (SMC)	150	71.1 (7.0)	23.3%	Community
Peavy et al., 2013 [93]	Subjective memory complaints (SMC)	39	78.5 (5.4)	Undisclosed	Clinic
Jessen et al., 2014 [60]	Subjective memory impairment (SMI) - *With concerns* - *Without concerns*	1061 *261* *800*	79.8 (3.5) *79.6 (3.4)* *79.8 (3.5)*	19.8% *20.7%* *18.8%*	Clinic
Kryscio et al., 2014 [56]	Subjective memory complaints (SMC)	531[a]	73.2 (7.4)[a]	30.3%[a]	Community
Mattsson et al., 2014 [54]	Subjective memory complaints (SMC)	68	72.0 (6.0)	30.0%	Community
Cherbuin et al., 2015 [51]	Subjective memory decline (SMD)	126	62.4 (1.5)[b]	19.6%[b]	Community
Hall et al., 2015 [94]	Subjective cognitive impairment (SCI)	231	67.9 (7.7)	40.0%	Clinic

[a] Data for total sample where SCD-specific data was not available
[b] Data for SCD at follow up only (regardless of baseline status or n)
[c] Data for total pooled SCD sample
[d] Data represents a purposefully matched sample of APOE+ to APOE-

Table 1 Continued

Study	SCD-Equivalent Classification	SCD *n*	SCD Mean Age (SD)	SCD % APOE-ε4	Sample Type
Hong et al., 2015 [59]	Subjective memory impairment (SMI)	129[c]	67.15 (7.8)[c]	29.5%[c]	Clinic
Krell-Roesch et al., 2015 [95]	Subjective cognitive impairment (SCI)	56	Range: 70-91[a]	51.0%[a]	Community
Lee et al., 2015 [47]	Subjective memory impairment (SMI)	26	66.3 (7.1)	50.0%[c]	Clinic
Risacher et al., 2015 [52]	Subjective memory concerns (SMC)	104	71.4 (5.5)	31.27%	Clinic
Snitz et al., 2015 [68]	Subjective cognitive decline (SCD)	14	68.1 (4.0)	30.8%	Clinic
Albers et al., 2016 [96]	Subjective cognitive concerns (SCC)	74	77.0 (0.9)	23.0%	Clinic
Fernández-Blázquez et al., 2016 [71]	Subjective cognitive decline (SCD) - *SCD* - *SCD-Plus*	423 *370* *53*	73.8 (3.6) *74.2 (3.8)* *73.3 (3.4)*	18.4% *16.7%* *29.4%*	Community
Sierra-Rio et al., 2016 [97]	Subjective cognitive decline (SCD)	55	66.7 (7.3)	25.5%	Clinic
Voevodskaya et al., 2016 [98]	Subjective cognitive decline (SCD)	49	70.7 (5.7)	71.0%	Clinic
Zwan et al., 2016 [57]	Subjective memory complaints (SMC)	168	73.0 (7)[a]	34.0%[a]	Community
Bridel et al., 2017 [99]	Subjective memory complaints (SMC)	20	60.3 (2.7)	50.0%	Clinic
Pařízková et al., 2017 [100]	Subjective cognitive decline (SCD)	46	69.1 (6.4)	14.0%	Clinic

[a] Data for total sample where SCD-specific data was not available
[b] Data for SCD at follow up only (regardless of baseline status or *n*)
[c] Data for total pooled SCD sample
[d] Data represents a purposefully matched sample of APOE+ to APOE-

Table 1 Continued

Study	SCD-Equivalent Classification	SCD n	SCD Mean Age (SD)	SCD % APOE-ε4	Sample Type
Dubois et al., 2018 [55]	Subjective memory complaints	318	76.0 (3.5)	20.0%	Mixed
Wirth et al., 2018 [101]	Subjective cognitive decline (SCD)	16	68.9 (7.3	19.0%	Clinic

[a] Data for total sample where SCD-specific data was not available
[b] Data for SCD at follow up only (regardless of baseline status or n)
[c] Data for total pooled SCD sample
[d] Data represents a purposefully matched sample of APOE+ to APOE-

Figure 1.1: Search protocol

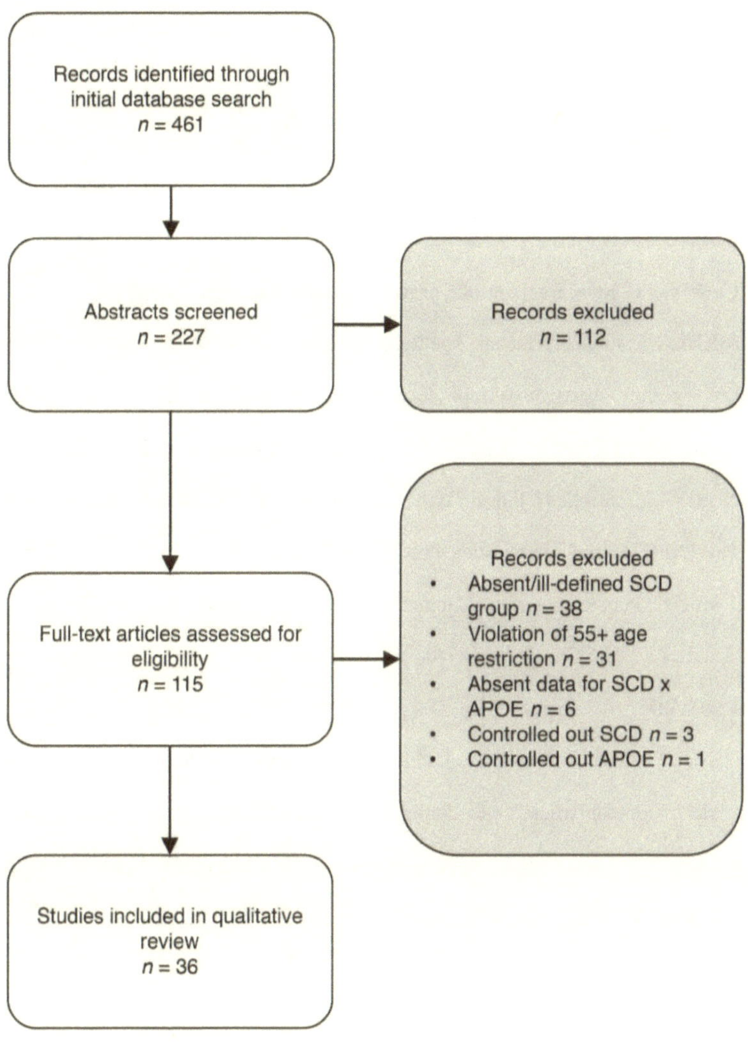

Appendix A: Search Protocol

Boolean Search Term

("subjective cognitive*" OR "subjective memory*" OR "cognitive complain*" OR "cognitive concern*" OR "memory complain*") AND ("APOE*" OR "apolipo*" OR "genetic" OR "genotype")

Delimiters by Database

CINAHL Complete. English language; Publication Type: "Journal Article", "Randomized Controlled Trial", "Research".

Cochrane Central Register of Controlled Trials. Language: "English".

MEDLINE. English; Human; Age Related: "Middle Aged: 45-64 years", "Middle Aged + Aged: 45 + years", "Aged: 65 + years", "Aged, 80 and over"; Publication Type: "Clinical Trial", "Clinical Trial, Phase I", "Clinical Trial, Phase II", "Clinical Trial, Phase III", "Clinical Trial, Phase IV", "Controlled Clinical Trial", "Journal Article", "Randomized Controlled Trial".

PsycINFO. English; Publication Type: "Peer Reviewed Journal"; Document Type: "Journal Article"; Population Group: "Human"; Age Groups: "Middle Age (40-64 yrs)", "Aged (65 yrs & older)", "Very Old (85 yrs & older)".

PubMED. Article types: "Clinical Study", "Clinical Trial", "Clinical Trial, Phase I", "Clinical Trial, Phase II", "Clinical Trial, Phase III", "Clinical Trial Phase IV", "Controlled Clinical Trial", "Journal Article", "Randomized Controlled Trial"; Text availability: "Full text"; Species: "Humans"; Ages: "Middle Aged: 45-64 years", "Middle Aged + Aged: 45 + years", "Aged: 65+ years", "80 and over: 80+ years".

Supplementary Materials: Excluded Articles

Absent/Ill-Defined SCD Group

- Blesa R, Adroer R, Santacruz P, Ascaso C, Tolosa E, Oliva R (1996) High apolipoprotein E ε4 allele frequency in age-related memory decline. *Ann. Neurol.* **39**, 548–551.

- Buckley R, Saling MM, Ames D, Rowe CC, Lautenschlager NT, Macaulay SL, Martins RN, Masters CL, O'Meara T, Savage G, Szoeke C, Villemagne VL, Ellis KA (2013) Factors affecting subjective memory complaints in the AIBL aging study: Biomarkers, memory, affect, and age. *Int. Psychogeriatrics* **25**, 1307–1315.

- Charidimou A, Ni J, Martinez-Ramirez S, Vashkevich A, Ayres A, Rosand J, Gurol EM, Greenberg SM, Viswanathan A (2016) Cortical superficial siderosis in memory clinic patients: Further evidence for underlying cerebral amyloid angiopathy. *Cerebrovasc. Dis.* **41**, 156–162.

- Chen Y, Denny KG, Harvey D, Farias ST, Mungas D, DeCarli C, Beckett L (2017) Progression from normal cognition to mild cognitive impairment in a diverse clinic-based and community-based elderly cohort. *Alzheimer's Dement.* **13**, 399–405.

- Clarnette RM (2001) Clinical characteristics of individuals with subjective memory loss in Western Australia: Results from a cross- sectional survey. **174**, 168–174.

- Collie A, Maruff P, Currie J (2002) Behavioral characterization of mild cognitive impairment. *J. Clin. Exp. Neuropsychol.* **24**, 720–733.

- Damian M, Hausner L, Jekel K, Richter M, Froelich L, Almkvist O, Boada M, Bullock R, De Deyn PP, Frisoni GB, Hampel H, Jones RW, Kehoe P, Lenoir H, Minthon L, Olde Rikkert MGM, Rodriguez G, Scheltens P, Soininen H, Spiru L, Touchon J, Tsolaki M, Vellas B, Verhey FRJ, Winblad B, Wahlund LO, Wilcock G, Visser PJ (2013) Single-domain amnestic mild cognitive impairment identified by cluster analysis predicts Alzheimer's disease in the european prospective DESCRIPA study. *Dement. Geriatr. Cogn. Disord.* **36**, 1–19.

- Derby CA, Burns LC, Wang C, Katz MJ, Zimmerman ME, L'italien G, Guo Z, Berman RM, Lipton RB (2013) Screening for predementia AD: Time-dependent operating characteristics of episodic memory tests. *Neurology* **80**, 1307–1314.

- Guaita A, Vaccaro R, Davin A, Colombo M, Vitali SF, Polito L, Abbondanza S, Valle E, Forloni G, Ferretti VV, Villani S (2015) Influence of socio-demographic features and apolipoprotein E ε4 expression on the prevalence of dementia and cognitive impairment in a population of 70 – 74-year olds: The InveCe.Ab study. *Arch. Gerontol. Geriatr.* **60**, 334–343.

- Harwood DG, Barker WW, Ownby RL, Mullan M, Duara R (2004) No association between subjective memory complaints and apolipoprotein E genotype in cognitively intact elderly. *Int. J. Geriatr. Psychiatry* **19**, 1131–1139.

- Heser K, Tebarth F, Wiese B, Eisele M, Bickel H, Köhler M, Mösch E, Weyerer S, Werle J, König H-H, Leicht H, Pentzek M, Fuchs A, Riedel-Heller SG, Luppa M, Prokein J, Scherer M, Maier W, Wagner M (2013) Age of major depression onset, depressive symptoms, and risk for subsequent dementia: Results of the German Study on Ageing, Cognition, and Dementia in primary care patients (AgeCoDe). *Psychol. Med.* **43**, 1597–610.

- Heun R, Kölsch H, Jessen F (2006) Risk factors and early signs of Alzheimer's disease in a family study sample: Risk of AD. *Eur. Arch. Psychiatry Clin. Neurosci.* **256**, 28–36.

- Horn MM, Kennedy KM, Rodrigue KM (2018) Association between subjective memory assessment and associative memory performance: Role of AD risk factors. *Psychol. Aging* **33**, 109–118.

- Jorm AF, Butterworth P, Anstey KJ, Christensen H, Easteal S, Maller J, Mather KA, Turakulov RI, Wen W, Sachdev P (2004) Memory complaints in a community sample aged 60-64 years: Associations with cognitive functioning, psychiatric symptoms, medical conditions, APOE genotype, hippocampus and amygdala volumes, and white-matter hyperintensities. *Psychol. Med.* **34**, 1495–506.

- Jungwirth S, Zehetmayer S, Bauer P, Weissgram S, Tragl KH, Fischer P (2009) Prediction of Alzheimer dementia with short neuropsychological instruments. *J. Neural Transm.* **116**, 1513–1521.

- Keegan AP, Paris D, Luis CA, Abdullah L, Ait-Ghezala G, Beaulieu-Abdelahad D, Pryor M, Chaykin J, Crynen G, Crawford F, Mullan M (2018) Plasma cytokine IL-6 levels and subjective cognitive decline: preliminary findings. *Int. J. Geriatr. Psychiatry* **33**, 358–363.

- Klimkowicz-Mrowiec A, Marona M, Wołkow P, Maruszak A, Styczynska M, Barcikowska M, Zekanowski C, Szczudlik A, Slowik A (2009) Interleukin-1 gene – 511 CT polymorphism and the risk of Alzheimer's disease in a Polish population. *Dement. Geriatr. Cogn. Disord.* **28**, 461–464.

- Laws SM, Clarnette RM, Taddei K, Martins G, Paton A, Almeida OP, Förstl H, Martins RN (2002) Association between the presenilin-1 mutation Glu318Gly and complaints of memory impairment. *Neurobiol. Aging* **23**, 55–58.

- Laws SM, Clarnette RM, Taddei K, Martins G, Paton A, Hallmayer J, Almeida OP, Groth DM, Gandy SE, Förstl H, Martins RN (2002) APOE- ε4 and APOE -491A polymorphisms in individuals with subjective memory loss. *Mol. Psychiatry* **7**, 768–75.

- Harwood DG, Barker WW, Ownby RL, Mullan M, Duara R (1999) Factors associated with depressive symptoms in non-demented community-dwelling elderly. **337**, 1131-1139.

- Lim YY, Laws SM, Villemagne VL, Pietrzak RH, Porter T, Ames D, Fowler C, Rainey-Smith S, Snyder PJ, Martins RN, Salvado O, Bourgeat P, Rowe CC, Masters CL, Maruff P (2016) Aβ-related memory decline in APOE ε4 noncarriers. *Neurology* **86**, 1635–1642.

- Mielke MM, Wiste HJ, Weigand SD, Knopman DS, Lowe VJ, Roberts RO, Geda YE, Swenson-Dravis DM, Boeve BF, Senjem ML, Vemuri P, Petersen RC, Jack Jr. CR (2012) Indicators of amyloid burden in a population-based study of cognitively normal elderly. *Neurology* **79**, 1570–1577.

- Mollica MA, Navarra J, Fernández-Prieto I, Olives J, Tort A, Valech N, Coll-Padrós N, Molinuevo JL, Rami L (2017) Subtle visuomotor difficulties in preclinical Alzheimer's disease. *J. Neuropsychol.* **11**, 56–73.

- Nicholas CR, Dowling NM, Racine AM, Clark LR, Berman SE, Koscik RL, Asthana S, Hermann B, Sager MA, Johnson SC (2017) Longitudinal assessment of self- and informant-subjective cognitive complaints in a sample of healthy late-middle aged adults enriched with a family history of Alzheimer's disease. *J. Int. Neuropsychol. Soc.* **23**, 617–626.

- Pekkala T, Hall A, Lötjönen J, Mattila J, Soininen H, Ngandu T, Laatikainen T, Kivipelto M, Solomon A (2017) Development of a late-life dementia prediction index with supervised machine learning in the population-based CAIDE study. *J. Alzheimer's Dis.* **55**, 1055–1067.

- Pietrzak RH, Lim YY, Ames D, Harrington K, Restrepo C, Martins RN, Rembach A, Laws SM, Masters CL, Villemagne VL, Rowe CC, Maruff P, Australian Imaging Biomarkers, Lifestyle (AIBL) Research Group (2015) Trajectories of memory decline in preclinical Alzheimer's disease: Results from the Australian Imaging, Biomarkers and Lifestyle flagship study of ageing. *Arch. Gerontol. Geriatr.* **36**, 1231–1238.

- Risacher SL, Kim S, Shen L, Nho K, Foroud T, Green RC, Petersen RC, Jack CR, Aisen PS, Koeppe RA, Jagust WJ, Shaw LM, Trojanowski JQ, Weiner MW, Saykin AJ (2013) The role of apolipoprotein E (APOE) genotype in early mild cognitive impairment (E-MCI). *Front. Aging Neurosci.* **5**, 1–12.

- Samieri C, Proust-Lima C, Glymour MM, Okereke OI, Amariglio RE, Sperling RA, Rentz DM, Grodstein F (2014) Subjective cognitive concerns, episodic memory, and the APOE ε4 allele. *Alzheimer's Dement.* **10**, 752–759.

- Stenset V, Hofoss D, Berstad AE, Negaard A, Gjerstad L, Fladby T (2008) White matter lesion subtypes and cognitive deficits in patients with memory impairment. *Dement. Geriatr. Cogn. Disord.* **26**, 424–431.

- Stenset V, Hofoss D, Johnsen L, Skinningsrud A, Berstad AE, Negaard A, Reinvang I, Gjerstad L, Fladby T (2008) White matter lesion severity is associated with reduced cognitive performances in patients with normal CSF Aβ42 levels. *Acta Neurol. Scand.* **118**, 373–378.

- Studer J, Donati A, Popp J, von Gunten A (2014) Subjective cognitive decline in patients with mild cognitive impairment and healthy older adults: Association with personality traits. *Geriatr. Gerontol. Int.* **14**, 589–595.

- Tanaka H, Ogata S, Omura K, Honda C, Kamide K, Hayakawa K (2015) Association between subjective memory complaints and depressive symptoms after adjustment for genetic and family environmental factors in a Japanese twin study. *Environ. Health Prev. Med.* **21**, 92–99.

- Tsuang D, Larson EB, Bowen J, McCormick W, Teri L, Nochlin D, Leverenz JB, Peskind ER, Lim a, Raskind M a, Thompson ML, Mirra SS, Gearing M, Schellenberg GD, Kukull W (1999) The utility of apolipoprotein E genotyping in the diagnosis of Alzheimer disease in a community-based case series. *Arch. Neurol.* **56**, 1489–95.

- van den Kommer TN, Bontempo DE, Comijs HC, Hofer SM, Dik MG, Piccinin AM, Jonker C, Deeg DJH, Johansson B (2009) Classification models for early identification of persons at risk for dementia in primary care: An evaluation in a sample aged 80 years and older. *Dement. Geriatr. Cogn. Disord.* **28**, 567–577.

- Vannini P, Hanseeuw B, Munro CE, Amariglio RE, Marshall GA, Rentz DM, Pascual-Leone A, Johnson KA, Sperling RA (2017) Hippocampal hypometabolism in older adults with memory complaints and increased amyloid burden. *Neurology* **88**, 1759–1767.

- Verlinden VJA, Van Der Geest JN, De Bruijn RFAG, Hofman A, Koudstaal PJ, Ikram MA (2016) Trajectories of decline in cognition and daily functioning in preclinical dementia. *Alzheimer's Dement.* **12**, 144–153.

- Weaver Cargin J, Collie A, Masters C, Maruff P (2008) The nature of cognitive complaints in healthy older adults with and without objective memory decline. *J. Clin. Exp. Neuropsychol.* **30**, 245–257.

Violation of 55+ Age Criteria

- Almkvist O, Tallberg I-M (2009) Cognitive decline from estimated premorbid status predicts neurodegeneration in Alzheimer's disease. *Neuropsychology* **23**, 117–124.

- Archer HA, MacFarlane F, Price S, Moore EK, Pepple T, Cutler D, Frost C, Fox NC, Rossor MN (2006) Do symptoms of memory impairment correspond to cognitive impairment: A cross sectional study of a clinical cohort. *Int. J. Geriatr. Psychiatry* **21**, 1206–1212.

- Bartres-Faz D, Junque C, Lopez-Alomar A, Valveny N, Moral P, Casamayor R, Salido A, Bel C, Clemente IC (2001) Neuropsychological and genetic differences between age-associated memory impairment and mild cognitive impairment entities. *J. Am. Geriatr. Soc.* **49**, 985–990.

- Bates KA, Sohrabi HR, Rodrigues M, Beilby J, Dhaliwal SS, Taddei K, Criddle A, Wraith M, Howard M, Martins G, Paton A, Mehta P, Foster JK, Martins IJ, Lautenschlager NT, Mastaglia FL, Laws SM, Gandy SE, Martins RN (2009) Association of cardiovascular factors and Alzheimer's disease plasma amyloid-β protein in subjective memory complainers. *J. Alzheimer's Dis.* **17**, 305–318.

- Boots EA, Schultz SA, Oh JM, Larson J, Edwards D, Cook D, Koscik RL, Dowling MN, Gallagher CL, Carlsson CM, Rowley HA, Bendlin BB, LaRue A, Asthana S, Hermann BP, Sager MA, Johnson SC, Okonkwo OC (2015) Cardiorespiratory fitness is associated with brain structure, cognition, and mood in a middle-aged cohort at risk for Alzheimer's disease. *Brain Imaging Behav.* **9**, 639–649.

- Caselli RJ, Chen K, Locke DEC, Lee W, Roontiva A, Bandy D, Fleisher AS, Reiman EM (2014) Subjective cognitive decline: Self and informant comparisons. *Alzheimer's Dement.* **10**, 93–98.

- Corder EH, Jelic V, Basun H, Lannfelt L, Valind S, Winblad B, Nordberg A (1997) No difference in cerebral glucose metabolism in patients with Alzheimer disease and differing apolipoprotein E genotypes. *Arch. Neurol.* **54**, 273–277.

- Enache D, Solomon A, Cavallin L, Kåreholt I, Kramberger MG, Aarsland D, Kivipelto M, Eriksdotter M, Winblad B, Jelic V (2016) CAIDE Dementia Risk Score and biomarkers of neurodegeneration in memory clinic patients without dementia. *Neurobiol. Aging* **42**, 124–131.

- Ercoli L, Siddarth P, Huang S-C, Miller K, Bookheimer SY, Wright BC, Phelps ME, Small GM (2006) Perceived loss of memory ability and cerebral metabolic decline in persons with the apolipoprotein E-IV genetic risk for Alzheimer disease. *Arch. Gen. Psychiatry* **63**, 442–448.

- Fladby T, Palhaugen L, Selnes P, Waterloo K, Brathen G, Hessen E, Almdahl IS, Arntzen KA, Auning E, Eliassen CF, Espenes R, Grambaite R, Grøntvedt GR, Johansen KK, Johnsen SH, Kalheim LF, Kirsebom BE, Muller KI, Nakling AE, Rongven A, Sando SB, Siafarikas N, Stav AL, Tecelao S, Timon S, Bekkelund SI, Aarsland D (2017) Detecting at-risk Alzheimer's disease cases. *J. Alzheimer's Dis.* **60**, 97–105.

- Geijselaers SLC, Aalten P, Ramakers IHGB, De Deyn PP, Heijboer AC, Koek HL, Olderikkert MGM, Papma JM, Reesink FE, Smits LL, Stehouwer CDA, Teunissen CE, Verhey FRJ, Van Der Flier WM, Biessels GJ (2017) Association of Cerebrospinal Fluid (CSF) Insulin with Cognitive Performance and CSF Biomarkers of Alzheimer's Disease. *J. Alzheimer's Dis.* **61**, 309–320.

- Gottfries J, Blennow K, Lehmann MW, Regland B, Gottfries C-G (2001) One-carbon metabolism and other biochemical correlates of cognitive impairment as visualized by principal component analysis. *J. Geriatr. Psychiatry Neurol.* **14**, 109–114.

- Kester MI, Goos JDC, Teunissen CE, Benedictus MR, Bouwman FH, Wattjes MP,

Barkhof F, Scheltens P, van der Flier WM (2014) Associations between cerebral small-vessel disease and Alzheimer disease pathology as measured by cerebrospinal fluid biomarkers. *JAMA Neurol.* **71**, 855.

- Lautenschlager NT, Cox KL, Flicker L, Foster JK, van Bockxmeer FM (2008) Effect of physical activity on cognitive function in older adults at risk for Alzheimer disease. **300**, 1027–1037.

- Lautenschlager NT, Wu JS, Laws SM, Almeida OP, Clarnette RM, Joesbury K, Wagenpfeil S, Martins G, Paton A, Gandy SE, Forstl H, Martins RN (2005) Neurological soft signs are associated with APOE genotype, age and cognitive performance. *J. Alzheimers Dis.* **7**, 325–330.

- Mandecka M, Budziszewska M, Barczak A, Pepłońska B, Chodakowska-Żebrowska M, Filipek-Gliszczyńska A, Nesteruk M, Styczyńska M, Barcikowska M, Gabryelewicz T (2016) Association between cerebrospinal fluid biomarkers for Alzheimer's disease, APOE genotypes and auditory verbal learning task in subjective cognitive decline, mild cognitive impairment, and Alzheimer's Disease. *J. Alzheimer's Dis.* **54**, 157–168.

- Mosconi L, De Santi S, Brys M, Tsui WH, Pirraglia E, Glodzik-Sobanska L, Rich KE, Switalski R, Mehta PD, Pratico D, Zinkowski R, Blennow K, de Leon MJ (2008) Hypometabolism and altered cerebrospinal fluid markers in normal apolipoprotein E E4 carriers with subjective memory complaints. *Biol. Psychiatry* **63**, 609–618.

- Nacmias B, Bessi V, Bagnoli S, Tedde A, Cellini E, Piccini C, Sorbi S, Bracco L (2008) KIBRA gene variants are associated with episodic memory performance in subjective memory complaints. *Neurosci. Lett.* **436**, 145–147.

- Rimajova M, Lenzo NP, Wu J-S, Bates KA, Campbell A, Dhaliwal SS, McCarthy M,

Rodrigues M, Paton A, Rowe C, Foster JK, Martins RN (2008) Fluoro-2-deoxy-D-glucose (FDG)-PET in APOE ε4 carriers in the Australian population. *J. Alzheimers Dis.* **13**, 137–146.

- Small GW, Chen ST, Komo S, Ercoli L, Bookheimer S, Miller K, Lavretsky H, Saxena S, Kaplan A, Dorsey D, Scott WK, Saunders AM, Haines JL, Roses AD, Pericak-Vance MA (1999) Memory self-appraisal in middle-aged and older adults with the apolipoprotein E-4 allele. *Am. J. Psychiatry* **156**, 1035–1038.

- Small GW, Chen ST, Komo S, Ercoli L, Miller K, Siddarth P, Kaplan A, Dorsey D, Lavretsky H, Saxena S, Bookheimer SY (2001) Memory self-appraisal and depressive symptoms in people at genetic risk for Alzheimer's disease. *Int J Geriatr Psychiatry* **16**, 1071–1077.

- Small GW, Mazziotta JC, Collins MT, Baxter LR, Phelps ME, Mandelkern MA, Kaplan A, La Rue A, Adamson CF, Chang L (1995) Apolipoprotein E type 4 allele and cerebral glucose metabolism in relatives at risk for familial Alzheimer disease. *Jama* **273**, 942–947.

- Small GW, Siddarth P, Silverman DHS, Ercoli LM, Miller KJ, Lavretsky H, Bookheimer SY, Huang S-C, Barrio JR, Phelps ME (2008) Cognitive and cerebral metabolic effects of celecoxib versus placebo in people with age-related memory loss: Randomized controlled study. *Am. J. Geriatr. Psychiatry* **16**, 999–1009.

- Sohrabi HR, Bates KA, Rodrigues M, Taddei K, Martins G, Laws SM, Lautenschlager NT, Dhaliwal SS, Foster JK, Martins RN (2009) The relationship between memory complaints, perceived quality of life and mental health in apolipoprotein E ε4 carriers and non-carriers. *J. Alzheimer's Dis.* **17**, 69–79.

- Solomon A, Leoni V, Kivipelto M, Besga A, Öksengård AR, Julin P, Svensson L, Wahlund LO, Andreasen N, Winblad B, Soininen H, Björkhem I (2009) Plasma levels of 24S-hydroxycholesterol reflect brain volumes in patients without objective cognitive impairment but not in those with Alzheimer's disease. *Neurosci. Lett.* **462**, 89–93.

- Stenset V, Johnsen L, Kocot D, Negaard A, Skinningsrud A, Gulbrandsen P, Wallin A, Fladby T (2006) Associations between white matter lesions, cerebrovascular risk factors, and low CSF Aß42. *Neurology* **67**, 830–3.

- Treves TA, Chapman J, Bornstein NM, Verchovsky R, Asherov A, Veschev IO, Klimovitzki S, Korczyn A (1996) APOE-ε4 in age-related memory complaints and Alzheimer's disease. **3**, 515–518.

- Wahlund LO, Julin P, Lannfelt L, Lindqvist J, Svensson L (1999) Inheritance of the ApoE ε4 allele increases the rate of brain atrophy in dementia patients. *Dement Geriatr Cogn Disord* **10**, 262–268.

- Wang X, Wang H, Li H, Li T, Yu X (2014) Frequency of the apolipoprotein e ε4 allele in a memory clinic cohort in Beijing: A naturalistic descriptive study. *PLoS One* **9**, 1–7 .

- Wehling E, Lundervold AJ, Standnes B, Gjerstad L, Reinvang I, Lobo A, Launer L, Fratiglioni L, Andersen K, Carlo A Di, Breteler M, Copeland J, Dartigues J, Jagger C, Martinez-Lage J, Soininen H, Hofman A, Morris J, Storandt M, Miller J, McKeel D, Price J, Rubin E, Berg L, Petersen R, Arnaiz E, Almkvist O, Ivnik R, Tangalos E, d LW, Winblad B, Petersen R, Koivisto K, Reinikainen K, Hanninen T, Vanhanen M, Helkala E, Mykkanen L, Laakso M, Pyorala K, Riekkinen P, Fisk J, Merry H, Rockwood K, Tervo S, Kivipelto M, Hanninen T, Vanhanen M, Hallikainen M, Mannermaa A, Soininen H, Raber J, Huang Y, Ashford JW, Farrer L, Cupples L, Haines J, Hyman B, Kukull W,

Mayeux R, Myers R, Pericak-Vance M, Risch N, vanDuijn C, Farlow M, He Y, Tekin S,
Xu J, Lane R, Charles H, Bondi M, Salmon D, Monsch A, Galasko D, Butters N, Klauber
M, Thal L, Saitoh T, Small B, Rosnick C, Fratiglioni L, Backman L, Caselli R, Reiman E,
Osborne D, Hentz J, Baxter L, Hernandez J, Alexander G, Mortensen E, Hogh P, Lind J,
Persson J, Ingvar M, Larsson A, Cruts M, Broeckhoven C Van, Adolfsson R, Backman L,
Nilsson L, Petersson K, Nyberg L, Greenwood P, Parasuraman R, Espeseth T,
Greenwood P, Reinvang I, Fjell A, Walhovd K, Westlye L, Wehling E, Lundervold A,
Rootwelt H, Parasuraman R, Gerdes L, Berr C, Wancata J, Ritchie K, Sundet K,
Lundervold A, Folstein M, Folstein S, McHugh P, Lezak M, Howieson D, Loring D,
Wechsler D, Delis D, Kramer J, Kaplan E, Ober B, Andersen R, Wechsler D, Reitan R,
Davidson L, Jensen A, Rohwer W, Benton A, Hamsher K, Kaplan E, Goodglass H,
Weintraub S, Frisoni G, Scheltens P, Galluzzi S, Nobili F, Fox N, Robert P, Soininen H,
Wahlund L, Waldemar G, Salmon E, Cohen J, Tierney M, Yao C, Kiss A, McDowell I,
Albert M, Moss M, Tanzi R, Jones K, Chey J, Kim J, Cho H, Cohen R, Small C, Lalonde
F, Friz J, Sunderland T, Lautenschlager N, Flicker S, Vasikaran S, Leedman P, Almeida
O, Petersen R, Smith G, Waring S, Ivnik R, Tangalos E, Kokmen E, Devanand D, Pelton
G, Zamora D, Liu X, Tabert M, Goodkind M, Scarmeas N, Braun I, Stern Y, Mayeux R,
Palmer B, Boone K, Lesser I, Wohl M, deRetrou J, Wenisch E, Chausson C, Dray F,
Faucounau V, Rigaud A, Caselli R, Osborne D, Reiman E, Hentz J, Barbieri C, Saunders
A, Hardy J, Graff-Radford N, Hall G, Alexander G, Borroni B, Archetti S, Agosti C,
Akkawi N, Brambilla C, Caimi L, Caltagirone C, DiLuca M, Padovani A (2007) APOE
status and its association to learning and memory performance in middle aged and older
Norwegians seeking assessment for memory deficits. *Behav. Brain Funct.* **3**, 57.

- Zill P, Bürger K, Behrens S, Hampel H, Padberg F, Boetsch T, Möller HJ, Ackenheil M,

Bondy B (2000) Polymorphisms in the α-2 macroglobulin gene in psychogeriatric patients. *Neurosci. Lett.* **294**, 69–72.

Absent Data for SCD x APOE

- Chatterjee P, Goozee K, Sohrabi HR, Shen K, Shah T, Asih PR, Dave P, ManYan C, Taddei K, Chung R, Zetterberg H, Blennow K, Martins RN (2018) Association of plasma neurofilament light chain with neocortical amyloid-β load and cognitive performance in cognitively normal elderly participants. *J. Alzheimer's Dis.* **63**, 1–9.

- Jessen F, Wiese B, Bickel H, Eiffländer-Gorfer S, Fuchs A, Kaduszkiewicz H, Köhler M, Luck T, Mösch E, Pentzek M, Riedel-Heller SG, Wagner M, Weyerer S, Maier W, van den Bussche H (2011) Prediction of dementia in primary care patients. *PLoS One* **6**, 1–10.

- Laske C, Sohrabi HR, Jasielec MS, Müller S, Koehler NK, Gräber S, Förster S, Drzezga A, Mueller-Sarnowski F, Danek A, Jucker M, Bateman RJ, Buckles V, Saykin AJ, Martins RN, Morris JC, Dominantly Inherited Alzheimer Network (DIAN) (2015) Diagnostic value of subjective memory complaints assessed with a single item in dominantly inherited Alzheimer's disease: Results of the DIAN study. *Biomed Res. Int.* **2015**, 1–7.

- Luck T, Riedel-Heller SG, Luppa M, Wiese B, Wollny A, Wagner M, Bickel H, Weyerer S, Pentzek M, Haller F, Moesch E, Werle J, Eisele M, Maier W, Van Den Bussche H, Kaduszkiewicz H (2009) Risk factors for incident mild cognitive impairment - results from the German Study on Ageing, Cognition and Dementia in Primary Care Patients (AgeCoDe). *Acta Psychiatr. Scand.* **121**, 260–272.

- Marini S, Bagnoli S, Bessi V, Tedde A, Bracco L, Sorbi S, Nacmias B (2011) Implication of serotonin-transporter (5-HTT) gene polymorphism in subjective memory complaints and mild cognitive impairment (MCI). *Arch. Gerontol. Geriatr.* **52**, 71–74.

- Pike KE, Ellis KA, Villemagne VL, Good N, Chételat G, Ames D, Szoeke C, Laws SM, Verdile G, Martins RN, Masters CL, Rowe CC (2011) Cognition and beta-amyloid in preclinical Alzheimer's disease: Data from the AIBL study. *Neuropsychologia* **49**, 2384–2390.

Controlled Out SCD

- Hua X, Ching CRK, Mezher A, Gutman BA, Hibar DP, Bhatt P, Leow AD, Jack CR, Bernstein MA, Weiner MW, Thompson PM (2016) MRI-based brain atrophy rates in ADNI phase 2: Acceleration and enrichment considerations for clinical trials. *Neurobiol. Aging* **37**, 26–37.

- Niti M, Yap KB, Kua EH, Ng TP (2009) APOE-ε4, depressive symptoms, and cognitive decline in Chinese older adults: Singapore Longitudinal Aging Studies. *Journals Gerontol. Ser. A Biol. Sci. Med. Sci.* **64A**, 306–311.

- Pietrzak RH, Lim YY, Neumeister A, Ames D, Ellis KA, Harrington K, Lautenschlager NT, Restrepo C, Martins RN, Masters CL, Villemagne VL, Rowe CC, Maruff P (2015) Amyloid-β, anxiety, and cognitive decline in preclinical Alzheimer disease: A multicenter, prospective cohort study. *JAMA Psychiatry* **72**, 284.

Controlled Out APOE

- Qian J, Wolters FJ, Beiser A, Haan M, Ikram MA, Karlawish J, Langbaum JB, Neuhaus JM, Reiman EM, Roberts JS, Seshadri S, Tariot PN, Woods BMC, Betensky RA, Blacker D (2017) APOE-related risk of mild cognitive impairment and dementia for prevention trials: An analysis of four cohorts. *PLoS Med.* **14**, 70–75.

Supplementary Materials: SCD Classification

Table 1.S1: Classification schemes for SCD and SCD-equivalent samples

Study	SCD-Equivalent Classification	SCD Classification Method
Dik et al., 2001 [8]	Memory complaints	"Do you have problems with your memory?" = 'Yes'
Stewart et al., 2001[65]	Subjective memory impairment (SMI)	*Geriatric Mental State Schedule* ≥4
Maruyama et al., 2004 [87]	Memory complaints	Self- or family-reported memory complaints
Lautenschlager et al., 2005 [88]	Subjective memory complaints (SMC)	"Do you have any difficulty with your memory?" = 'Yes'
Jessen et al., 2007 [64]	Subjective memory impairment (SMI)	"Do you feel like your memory is becoming worse?" = 'Yes, this worries me' or 'Yes, but this does not worry me' Endorsed little to no impairment on questions derived from *Subjective Memory Decline Scale*
Chételat et al., 2010 [53]	Subjective cognitive impairment (SCI)	"Do you have any difficulty with your memory?" = 'Yes'
Rowe et al., 2010 [58]	Subjective memory complaints (SMC)	"Do you have any difficulty with your memory?" = 'Yes'
Striepens et al., 2010 [89]	Subjective memory impairment (SMI)	Self- and informant-reported memory impairment Onset of SMI in last 10 years
Watfa et al., 2010 [49]	Subjective memory complaints (SMC)	Revised French version (26-item) *McNair Scale* >15
Bartley et al., 2011 [48]	Subjective memory complaints (SMC)	"Do you feel like your memory or thinking is becoming worse?" = 'Yes and this worries me' or 'Yes, but this does not worry me'
Fortea at al., 2011 [90]	Subjective memory complaints (SMC)	Presented with subjective memory complaints
Norberg et al., 2011 [91]	Subjective cognitive impairment (SCI)	Presented with memory concerns

Table S1 continued

Study	SCD-Equivalent Classification	SCD Classification Method
Stewart et al., 2011 [50]	Subjective memory impairment (SMI)	Question re: habitual forgetfulness during daily activities = 'Yes'* Question re: difficulties remembering recent new information = 'Yes'*
Striepens et al., 2011 [46]	Subjective memory impairment (SMI)	Self- and informant-reported memory impairment Onset of SMI in last 10 years
Smith et al., 2012 [92]	Memory complaints	Self-reported memory complaints at baseline
Verdile et al., 2012 [63]	Subjective memory complaints (SMC)	"Do you have difficulties with your memory" = 'Yes'**
Peavy et al., 2013 [93]	Subjective memory complaints (SMC)	Question re: problems with memory representing a change from previous abilities = 'Yes'
Jessen et al., 2014 [60]	Subjective memory impairment (SMI)	"Do you feel like your memory is becoming worse?" = 'Yes, this worries me' or 'Yes, but this does not worry me'
Kryscio et al., 2014 [56]	Subjective memory complaints (SMC)	Self-reported SMC
Mattsson et al., 2014 [54]	Subjective memory complaints (SMC)	*Alzheimer's Disease Assessment Scale – cognitive subscale*
Cherbuin et al., 2015 [51]	Subjective memory decline (SMD)	Do you feel you can remember things as well as you used to?" = 'No'
Hall et al., 2015 [94]	Subjective cognitive impairment (SCI)	Self-reported cognitive complaints

* Stewart R, Dufouil C, Godin O, Ritchie K, Maillard P, Delcroix N, Crivello F, Mazoyer B, Tzourio C (2008) Neuroimaging correlates of subjective memory deficits in a Community population. *Neurology* **70**, 1601–1607.

** Ellis KA, Bush AI, Darby D, De Fazio D, Foster J, Hudson P, Lautenschlager NT, Lenzo N, Martins RN, Maruff P, Masters C, Milner A, Pike K, Rowe C, Savage G, Szoeke C, Taddei K, Villemagne V, Woodward M, Ames D, Acosta O, Ames J, Agarwal M, Bahar-Fuchs A, Baxendale D, Bechta-Metti K, Bevage C, Bevege L, Bourgeat P, Brown B, Bush A, Clarnette R, Cowie T, Crowley K, Currie A, El-Sheikh D, Ellis K, Dickinson K, Farrow M, Faux N, Fripp J, Fowler C, Gupta V, Jones G, Khoo J, Killedar A, Killeen N, Tae WK, Kotsopoulos E, Lachovitzki R, Lautenschlager N, Li QX, Liang X, Lucas K, Lui J, Martins G, Montague C, Moore L, Muir A, O'Halloran C, O'Keefe G, Panayiotou A, Paton A, Paton J, Peiffer J, Pejoska S, Pertile K, Porter L, Price R, Raniga P, Rees G, Rembach A, Rimajova M, Robins P, Ronsisvalle E, Rumble R, Rodrigues M, Salvado O, Sach J, Samuel M, Sittironnarit G, Taddei T, Trivedi D, Trounson B, Tsikkos M, Walker S, Ward V, Yastrubetskaya O (2009) The Australian Imaging, Biomarkers and Lifestyle (AIBL) study of aging: Methodology and baseline characteristics of 1112 individuals recruited for a longitudinal study of Alzheimer's disease. *Int. Psychogeriatrics* **21**, 672–687.

Table S1 continued

Study	SCD-Equivalent Classification	SCD Classification Method
Hong et al., 2015 [59]	Subjective memory impairment (SMI)	"Do you feel your memory is impaired" = 'Yes'
Krell-Roesch et al., 2015 [95]	Subjective cognitive impairment (SCI)	First item of *Memory Frequency Questionnaire* <7
Lee et al., 2015 [47]	Subjective memory impairment (SMI)	Sustained subjective memory complaints
Risacher et al., 2015 [52]	Subjective memory concerns (SMC)	Total score of first 12 items from *Cognitive Change Index* (selected items from a larger compilation of measures) >16
Snitz et al., 2015 [68]	Subjective cognitive decline (SCD)	Presented with memory/thinking concerns
Albers et al., 2016 [96]	Subjective cognitive concerns (SCC)	Concerns about cognition
Fernández-Blázquez et al., 2016 [71]	Subjective cognitive decline (SCD)	'Yes' to any of the following: "Are you easily distracted?" "Do you get lost in familiar surroundings or have trouble finding your way when driving?" "Do you often forget recent information or events?" "Do you often forget autobiographical information?" "Do you have trouble recognizing objects or faces?" "Do you have word finding difficulties for people's names or common words?" "Do you understand simple verbal and written instructions?" "Do you have difficulty driving, managing finances or planning daily activities?" "Do you have difficulties sequencing movements (e.g., taking the necessary steps to prepare a bath)?"

(continued)

Table S1 continued

Study	SCD-Equivalent Classification	SCD Classification Method
Fernández-Blázquez et al., 2016 [71] (*cont'd*)		SCD scale (ordinal, 0-3) total score >1: "How do you perceive your memory in comparison with that of others your age?" "How do you perceive your memory today compared with your young adulthood?" "Do you perceive your memory today is worse than compared with ten years ago?" "Do you perceive your memory today is worse than compared with one year ago?"
Sierra-Rio et al., 2016 [97]	Subjective cognitive decline (SCD)	Presented with self- or family-reported cognitive concerns
Voevodskaya et al., 2016 [98]	Subjective cognitive decline (SCD)	Presented with cognitive complaints
Zwan et al., 2016 [57]	Subjective memory complaints (SMC)	"Do you have any difficulty with your memory?" = 'Yes'
Bridel et al., 2017 [99]	Subjective memory complaints (SMC)	Results of clinical examination normal No psychiatric diagnosis Presence of cognitive complaints
Pařízková et al., 2017 [100]	Subjective cognitive decline (SCD)	Self-reported memory complaints
Dubois et al., 2018 [55]	Subjective memory complaints	Presented with memory complaints
Wirth et al., 2018 [101]	Subjective cognitive decline (SCD)	Self-reported cognitive concerns

Chapter 2: Research Methods

Introduction

The following chapter presents a comprehensive description of the methods and measures employed for this book study. Given that our variables of interest, recruitment, sample, and data collection procedures were shared between our studies, it was considered useful to present these separately. The specific analyses used for our studies are presented in their respective chapters.

Methods

Primary Classification Variables of Interest

Subjective cognitive decline (SCD. A substantial body of work has demonstrated that cognitive complaints and self-reported declines are typical of the aging experience and, as such, may provide limited benefit for predicting an individuals' cognitive trajectory. Conversely, it has been suggested that *concerns* about cognitive decline are significantly more predictive of later declines (Jessen et al., 2014). The Subjective Cognitive Decline Initiative (SCD-I) Working Group's criteria for SCD that is high risk for AD (SCD *Plus*; Jessen et al., 2014) explicitly lists having concerns associated with SCD as a key risk factor. Other items that may increase the likelihood of preclinical AD among those with SCD are reporting subjective declines in memory versus other cognitive domains, SCD onset within five years, being older than 60 years of age at the time of SCD onset, and feeling that one's (cognitive) performance is worse than same-aged peers. Additional factors that may reinforce the likelihood of preclinical AD among those with SCD is informant corroboration of cognitive declines, presence of the APOE ε4 allele, and other AD-consistent biomarker evidence. Thus, the classification of SCD endorsement in the current study was informed by and corroborating studies (Jessen et al., 2020; Jessen et al., 2014; Rabin et al., 2015).

Subtle cognitive decline (subtle CD). In addition to the classification of SCD based on self-identification, participants were classified as healthy controls or as demonstrating subtle CD based on their neuropsychological test performance. We applied Edmonds and colleagues' criteria for subtle CD with few amendments to better suit the large battery used in this study (Edmonds et al., 2015). Specifically, Edmonds et al. administered an abbreviated battery of six tests divided equally across three cognitive domains (i.e., two tests per domain). Their criteria state that individuals with a single score >1 SD below age-normed mean distributed across each of two neuropsychological domains may be assumed to have declined from their previous/expected level of ability and, consequently, were considered to demonstrate subtle CD. In contrast, individuals with more than one low score within a domain or with a single low score in each of the three domains were considered to have probable MCI.

Previous work demonstrates the high probability – even typicality – of scores >1 SD below age-normed means even in healthy individuals (Binder, Iverson, & Brooks, 2009). Given the increased likelihood of familywise error due to the greater number of tests administered in the current study, we retained Edmonds et al.'s inclusion criteria for subtle CD but discarded their frequency-based criterion for exclusion (i.e., MCI) in favor of a percentage-based criterion (i.e., if >50% of an individual's scores within a given cognitive domain are >1 standard deviation below the age-normative mean, they are considered to have MCI and were ineligible for inclusion). We believe this amendment stays true to the intent of Edmonds et al.'s definition while allowing for its application to a more comprehensive battery.

APOE ε4 genotype. APOE ε4 has been consistently identified as a risk factor for conversion to AD and vascular dementia (Allan & Ebmeier, 2011; Chen et al., 2016; Jiang et al., 2016; Liu et al., 2016; Mata et al., 2014; Pink et al., 2015; Prestia et al., 2015). APOE ε4 carriers have been estimated to have approximately three times greater risk of developing AD, while double allele carriers are estimated to be approximately 15 times more likely than the general population to develop AD (Farrer et al., 1997). With respect to SCD, a recent review found that APOE ε4 does not impact the development of SCD (broadly defined), but that SCD and APOE ε4 confer independent and interacting risk for conversion to an objectively cognitively impaired state (Ali et al., 2018). Given the relationship between SCD, APOE ε4, and AD-consistent neuropathology, the APOE ε4 genotype may provide crucial insight into risk for cognitive decline among those with SCD and may contextualize otherwise ambiguous evidence provided through other approaches. It is for exactly this reason that both the SCD Plus guidelines for high-risk SCD (Jessen et al., 2014) and NIA preclinical AD criteria (Jack et al., 2018) encourage the collection of biomarker data to supplement neuropsychological test scores when assessing cognitive risk.

Participants

Eligibility. Eligible participants were adults >65 years of age living independently in British Columbia, Canada. In line with Jessen and coworkers' criteria of no cognitive or functional impairment (Jessen et al., 2014), eligible participants had never received a diagnosis related to cognitive impairment or any specific neurological disorder (e.g., dementia, stroke, etc.) and were cognitively and functionally intact (i.e., able to live independently and perform activities of daily living). Potential participants were considered to have probable MCI and, consequently, were excluded from analyses if they a) achieved a z-score <2.00 on the Memory and Aging Telephone Screen (Rabin et al., 2007); b) achieved a score <24 on the MMSE-2 cognitive screening measure, c) achieved a score <8 on the Lawton-Brody IADL scale (Graf, 2008) , or d) scored >1 standard deviation below the age-normative mean across the majority of neuropsychological tests loading onto any single cognitive domain (Edmonds et al., 2015).

SCD group classification. Participants' SCD endorsement was determined by first exploring whether they had noticed any cognitive changes/declines within the past five years and then following up with a single query: "Are your cognitive changes concerning to you (e.g., more than you would expect compared to others your age)?". Participants responding "yes" to this query were classified as SCD endorsers.

Subtle CD group classification. Participants were categorized as healthy controls (absent subtle CD) or as evidencing subtle CD based on their aggregate performance across a neuropsychological assessment battery.

Recruitment. Study recruitment was approached through multiple avenues. Recruitment posters advertising the study as an investigation into experiences of aging and cognition were posted at community centres, libraries, and family doctors' offices throughout Southern Vancouver Island, British Columbia, Canada. Letters including our advertisement materials were sent to the offices of neuropsychologists, family physicians, and older adult service providers (e.g., recreational programs) in the Capital Regional District and Greater Vancouver Regional District that we were unable to visit in person. Our advertisements were also posted throughout the University of Victoria and on its digital advertising platform. Several research recruitment talks were given at University of Victoria-sponsored research events and local older adult programs. Aside from the direct recruitment activities undertaken by the research team, several partner organizations assisted with the distribution of our advertising materials. The University of Victoria Institute on Aging and Lifelong Health sent the advertisements and additional study information to their network of older adults in the local community as did the University of Victoria Retirees' Association.

Measures and Materials

Screening measures. Participants completed several screening measures during an initial telephone screening interview and the neuropsychological assessment. Screening items were also included in a demographic questionnaire probing medical and mental health history. Measures created by the authors or openly available are presented in Appendix B.

Demographics and health history. A demographics and physical/mental health history questionnaire was created for use in this study. Questionnaire items queried general demographic details (e.g., age, sex, education, etc.), presence of physical health adversities known to impact cognitive functioning, previous and/or current mental health adversities, family history of cognitive disorder, and previous genetic testing experience. In particular, items pertaining to age and history of neurological disorder were used as screening items.

Lawton-Brody Instrumental Activities of Daily Living Scale (IADL; Graf, 2008). This eight-item scale provides insight into the ability of older adults to complete common daily activities independently. This was used as a proxy measure, in combination with others, to determine whether potential participants were cognitively and functionally intact. The IADL scale has been found to have a high inter-rater reliability with the Physical Self-Maintenance Scale ($r=.85$) as well as significant correlations with the Behavior and Adjustment rating scales, the Physical Status scales, and the Mental Status Questionnaire (Hokoishi et al., 2001).

Memory and Aging Telephone Screen (MATS; Rabin et al., 2007). The MATS was embedded in our demographic questionnaire. In addition to being used as a gross cognitive screening measure to determine eligibility alongside the MMSE-2, MATS responses were used to determine SCD group eligibility.

Mini-Mental State Exam, Second Edition (MMSE-2: SV; Folstein, Folstein, 2009). The MMSE-2 is considered a "gold standard" clinical screening measure for dementia or cognitive impairment. It is a key measure used in dementia diagnosis and, when used as part of a more comprehensive workup, can help to differentiate healthy individuals from those with varying degrees of objective cognitive impairment. The MMSE-2 was used to rule out those with probable objective cognitive decline.

Self-report cognitive measures.

Cognitive Change Index (CCI; Saykin et al., 2006). The CCI measures individuals' perceptions of cognitive change over time across several cognitive domains, including memory, language, and executive functioning. The CCI scores correspond relatively well with objective test performance (Rattanabannakit et al., 2016). High scores on the CCI indicate a greater degree of perceived cognitive change. Although the CCI's content clearly overlaps with perceived cognitive change, it is less clear whether it reflects the concern aspect of SCD.

Measurement of Everyday Cognition, select subscales (ECog; Farias et al., 2008). The full ECog measures self-reported cognitive ability relative to same-aged peers across six domains, including memory, language, visuospatial ability, planning, organization, and divided attention. The ECog has excellent test-retest reliability ($r=.82$) as well as strong convergent and discriminative validity when compared to other measures. For efficiency, the language and visuospatial ability subscales of the ECog were excluded in the current study. Specifically, the language section was considered unduly burdensome for older adults within the context of the larger assessment battery and its redundancy with screening questions (MATS) related to perceived word-finding difficulties. The visuospatial ability section was excluded as we did not perform any corroborative objective testing of visuospatial ability within our neuropsychological assessment. Thus, participants were only administered memory, planning, organization, and divided attention subscale items. Low scores on the ECog indicate worse functioning relative to same-aged peers, whereas high scores indicate better functioning relative to same-aged peers. The ECog is a commonly used measure in SCD studies and was considered a valuable inclusion in our analyses given our greater goal of identifying viable screening measures or items.

Memory and Aging Telephone Screen (MATS; Rabin et al., 2007). In addition to being used as a gross cognitive screening measure to determine eligibility alongside the MMSE-2, MATS responses were used to determine whether participants endorsed self-perceived changes in word-finding ability. Although word-finding challenges are typical of normative cognitive aging, declines in this area are commonly reported causes for distress among older adults. As such, it was deemed relevant to include the endorsement of word-finding declines in the regression analyses.

Self-report mood/mental health measures.

Adult Manifest Anxiety Scale, elderly version (AMAS-E; Reynolds, Richmond, Lowe, 2003). The AMAS has been found to be temporally stable, to have moderate to good correlation with other established measures (Lowe & Raad, 2006), and to be invariant with gender (Lowe & Reynolds, 2006). All forms of the AMAS include a validity scale which may provide insight into participants' openness to endorsing symptoms. The AMAS-E specifically contains subscales dedicated to worry/oversensitivity, physiological anxiety, and fear of aging in adults 60 years of age and older. The inclusion of the AMAS-E was key in our investigation of SCD and subtle CD. Anxiety has been consistently linked to the endorsement of SCD (e.g., Hill et al., 2016; Tandetnik et al., 2017). The role of anxiety in subtle CD remains unclear.

Geriatric Depression Scale, short form (GDS; Yesavage et al., 1982). The GDS is designed to reflect the unique presentation of depression in older adults, controlling for physical symptoms and health adversities. The GDS has been shown to have predictive validity in terms of quality of life, independent activities of daily living, and depressive mood, and has proven reliable with older adult populations (Cronbach's α=0.90). The GDS was included as it has been shown to influence self-reported cognitive functioning and concern (Tomita et al., 2014).

UCLA Loneliness Scale (Russell, Peplau, & Ferguson, 1978). In light of recent work demonstrating the unique accelerating effect of loneliness on cognitive decline (Donovan et al., 2017), it was considered important to include a measure of this variable. Factor analysis has shown UCLA Loneliness Scale outcomes to be invariant with age and to be highly internally consistent (Ausín, Muñoz, Martín, Pérez-Santos, & Castellanos, 2019).

Neuropsychological assessment. The neuropsychological test battery was designed to closely parallel the Uniform Data Set used in the large-scale Alzheimer's Disease Neuroimaging Initiative (ADNI) study (Weintraub et al., 2018). Lower than expected performance on neuropsychological measures was used to classify individuals as healthy controls or as demonstrating subtle CD.

Boston Naming Test, second edition (BNT; Kaplan, Goodglass, & Weintraub, 2000). The BNT is a measure of confrontation naming that is sensitive to disruptions in language. The BNT (or an abbreviated version) is commonly included in Alzheimer's research batteries (e.g., CERAD), as it has been shown to be sensitive to overall cognitive dysfunction (Mast & Gerstenecker, 2010).

California Verbal Learning Test, Second Edition (CVLT-2; Delis, Kramer, Kaplan, & Ober, 2000). The CVLT-2 measures verbal learning, retention, recall, and recognition. It further provides insight into executive functions, such as self-monitoring, inhibition (proneness to interference), and effort. Individuals with AD and other forms of objective cognitive impairment demonstrate clear and well-documented patterns of performance on the CVLT-2, making it an excellent diagnostic tool for objective cognitive decline (Gifford et al., 2015; Lezak, Howieson, Bigler, & Tranel, 2012).

Controlled Oral Word Association Test (COWAT; Ivnik et al., 1996). The COWAT is a test of verbal fluency, which includes aspects of executive functioning, word retrieval and processing speed (Lezak et al., 2012). As such, COWAT performance is sensitive to memory and prefrontal/executive deficits. Verbal fluency is not only sensitive to MCI, but the specific pattern of poor performance has been shown effective for differentiating specific pathologies (Price et al., 2012; Weakley, Schmitter-Edgecombe, & Anderson, 2013).

Golden Stroop Test (Stroop; Ivnik et al., 1996). The Stroop test provides insight into various cognitive functions, including processing speed, simple attention, word generation, and executive inhibition. Individuals with objective cognitive dysfunction, such as those with MCI and AD, have been found to perform more poorly than healthy controls on the inhibition task in particular (Bélanger, Belleville, & Gauthier, 2010).

Test of Practical Judgment (TOP-J; Rabin et al., 2007). The TOP-J is a measure designed to assess individuals' safety awareness and behaviours, problem-solving, and ability to navigate common daily activities. Owing to its' prefrontal/executive-loaded nature, the TOP-J has been shown to differentiate those with MCI, AD, and other objective cognitive impairment from cognitively intact individuals (Rabin et al., 2009). What is more, in the case that individuals are found to suffer from objective cognitive impairment, the TOP-J may provide insight into their relative safety in the community.

Trailmaking Test (TMT; Ivnik, Malec, Smith, Tangalos, & Petersen, 1996). Trailmaking Test A provides insight into simple attention, whereas Trailmaking Test B provides insight into selective attention, inhibition, and executive switching. Trailmaking Test B has been used to identify late-stage Alzheimer's disease and other prefrontal lobe dysfunction (Rapp & Reischies, 2005).

Wechsler Adult Intelligence Scale, fourth edition: Digit Span subtest (DS; Wechsler & Psychological Corporation, 2008). Digit span is a commonly used test in both clinical and research settings. Digit span-forward is a test of simple attention while digit span backward measures working memory. There is evidence that digit span is sensitive to MCI and may be sensitive to cognitive impairment among those with subjective memory complaints (Kurt, Yener, & Oguz, 2011). Analysis of reliable digit span may also be used as a measure of effort.

Wechsler Advanced Clinical Solution for the WAIS-IV and WMS-IV: Test of Premorbid Function (TOPF; Wechsler, 2008). The TOPF is commonly used in clinical and research settings to estimate premorbid cognitive ability based on demographic factors and performance on tasks insensitive to cognitive dysfunction (Wechsler, 2008). In the absence of comprehensive intelligence testing, the TOPF provides an estimate of individuals' baseline general intellectual ability. This is largely determined by education and socioeconomic status.

Wechsler Memory Scale, fourth edition: Logical Memory subtest (LM; Wechsler & Psychological Corporation, 2008). In contrast to the CVLT-2, which assesses memory for non-contextual verbal information, the LM measures the influence of organization, meaning, and context on learning, retention, and recall.

Wechsler Memory Scale, fourth edition: Visual reproduction subtest (VR; Wechsler & Psychological Corporation, 2008). VM assesses individuals' learning and memory for non-verbal information. This test also provides opportunity for qualitative observation of fine motor functioning and frank visual disturbance.

Genetic sample collection. To obtain participants' APOE ε4 status, the Oragene OG-500 DNA saliva collection kit, mailable tube format, was used to obtain saliva samples from each participant. Oragene PrepIT L2P was used as a reagent for DNA extraction.

Procedures

Consent. Preceding the telephone eligibility screening, verbal consent was obtained from all participants be obtained. Each individual was informed of the purposes of the study and had the various data collection activities described to them. Upon commencement of in-person data collection, participants were provided hard-copy consent forms with a greater degree of detail regarding the study aims, activities, and contact details of various research team members. Consent was discussed and participants were provided an opportunity to ask any questions. Consent was reviewed at the beginning of each data collection session. Consent forms may be found in Appendix A.

Data Collection. The study procedures were approved by the University of Victoria Human Research Ethics Board and all activities were conducted in accordance with the Declaration of Helsinki. Data collection (excluding the initial telephone eligibility screening) was distributed over three days, though several participants opted to divide these activities across additional days due to fatigue or time constraints. Data collection activities were completed in the sequence by each participant.

Day 0: Telephone screening interview. Following recruitment, participants participated in a telephone eligibility screening interview with either the Principal Investigator or a trained Research Assistant. As part of this initial telephone screen, participants were administered the demographics questionnaire, the MATS, and the IADL scale. This screening interview took approximately 45 minutes.

Day 1: Self-report measures and neuropsychological assessment. Participants were administered a packet containing the GDS, AMAS-E, UCLA Loneliness Scale, subscales of the ECog, and CCI. This portion of the session typically took 20-30 minutes and was followed by a brief break if desired. Following completion of the self-report measures, participants were administered the full neuropsychological assessment battery. Again, breaks were provided as necessary. Cognitive-neuropsychological testing took approximately two hours for most participants.

Day 2: Qualitative interview and saliva sampling. Day 2 was typically scheduled within one week of Day 1. Individuals participated in a semi-structured one-hour interview regarding their experiences with age-related cognitive change and their concerns regarding the course and potential outcome of these changes. This interview was conducted in a manner consistent with directed content analysis (Hsieh & Shannon, 2005). The interview schedule is presented in Appendix C. It should be noted that the prepared scheduled provided a foundation for the interviews but was not restrictive. Deviations from the presented content were permitted and encouraged as considered fit by the Principal Investigator or participants. As additional cases and data became available, certain items that were found to be saturated were deemphasized during subsequent interviews. Each interview was recorded to ensure accurate transcription and field notes were taken immediately after the completion of interviews to allow the Principal Investigator to better account for observations, personal assumptions, biases, and areas for follow up during member check. Interviews took a maximum of one hour.

Upon completion of the interview, participants were removed to a sterile area for biological sample collection. Saliva sample collection was conducted in line with approved Biosafety protocols and Standard Operating Procedures. Participants were handed an empty sample vial and asked to deposit their sample into the vial independently. Saliva samples were then collected by the Principal Investigator, coded, and stored for delivery to an external genotyping lab. Once processed, saliva samples were destroyed at the lab.

Member check and debrief. Within four weeks of the testing/interview session, the Principal Investigator emailed each participant a summary of main points (e.g., reported areas of strength, decline, concerns, etc.) derived from their transcribed interview data. Following receipt of their summaries, participants arranged a telephone follow up. After discussing the summaries, revisions were made to the extent that participants chose to elaborate, correct, or change their reports. Once confirmed as an accurate representation of their experiences, the resulting summaries were included as part of participants' qualitative data. Member check conversations typically took 15 minutes or less. Following completion of the member check, participants were debriefed as to the more specific aims of the study and how their data was to be used. A debriefing script is presented in Appendix D.

Compensation. Participants were provided a $10 honorarium for their participation in each data collection session.

Data Preparation

Quantitative data. Self-report and cognitive-neuropsychological measures were scored by the Principal Investigator, who is trained in the administration and interpretation of these tools. Ensuing raw and whole scores were entered into a database using SPSS statistical software, Version 27.

Qualitative data and procedural rigour. Each participants' interview and member check was recorded digitally. These recorded discussions were transcribed by two trained Research Assistants independently. The resulting transcripts were then combined by the Principal

Investigator to create a single record. Disagreements between the transcripts were resolved by the Principal Investigator with reference to the original audio file.

Various methods were used to optimize the procedural rigour of the qualitative data collection and analyses. Guiding principles were derived primarily from Lincoln and Guba's evaluative criteria for qualitative validity (1985) and Creswell and Miller's validation strategies (Creswell & Miller, 2000). Several methods for establishing credibility were employed. Qualitative data collection was conducted via interview, which is arguably the most credible method due to the individual nature of the data collected. Reflexivity, the continuous awareness and analysis of the interviewer-interviewee dynamic and researcher bias, was also be employed heavily throughout the data collection and analysis processes. The Principal Investigator maintained comprehensive notes during and following interviews regarding participant behaviours, personal assumptions, and impressions. These notes were referred to and biases accounted for during data analysis. Information disconfirming the Principal Investigators initial conclusions was specifically sought and considered in order to manage his potential biases. Finally, the member check was conducted over the phone to ensure that the data reflected the participants' experiences with aging and cognitive change rather than the Principal Investigators interpretations (Krefting, 1991). Triangulation between qualitative reports, informant reports, and genetic vulnerabilities was attempted but was ultimately unsuccessful due to our low n of informants and low representation of APOE ε4-positive genotype

To combat any potential violations of dependability (reliability), all research activities were recorded and dated. With respect to confirmability (objectivity), the Principal Investigator established an audit trail of all research activities, materials, and data. Further, transcription by several parties helped to ensure that interviewer bias exerted a minimal impact on the transcripted data. Categorization of qualitative experiences – particularly, those relating to change within given cognitive-neuropsychological domains – were peer reviewed by a co-author and registered clinical neuropsychologist. Theme- and category-level findings were presented with the support of relevant transcript excerpts.

The transferability of our findings is more difficult to establish. Challenges to transferability may arise in the form of selection bias. Specifically, there is potential that individuals who were more socially engaged, more willing/able to participant in research, and who may have a higher degree of confidence in their cognitive functioning may have been over-represented in our studies. Further older adults in southern Vancouver Island are known to be often relatively highly educated, financially secure, and physically healthy. As a result, our findings may represent the local population well but may not generalize to a broader, more diverse older adult population.

References

Ali, J. I., Smart, C. M., & Gawryluk, J. R. (2018). Subjective cognitive decline and APOE E4: A systematic review. *Journal of Alzheimer's Disease, 65*(1), 303–320.

Allan, C. L., & Ebmeier, K. P. (2011). The influence of ApoE4 on clinical progression of dementia: a meta-analysis. *International Journal of Geriatric Psychiatry, 26*(5), 520–526. https://doi.org/10.1002/gps.2559

Ausín, B., Muñoz, M., Martín, T., Pérez-Santos, E., & Castellanos, M. Á. (2019). Confirmatory factor analysis of the Revised UCLA Loneliness Scale (UCLA LS-R) in individuals over 65. *Aging and Mental Health, 23*(3), 345–351. https://doi.org/10.1080/13607863.2017.1423036

Bélanger, S., Belleville, S., & Gauthier, S. (2010). Inhibition impairments in Alzheimer's disease, mild cognitive impairment and healthy aging: Effect of congruency proportion in a Stroop task. *Neuropsychologia, 48*(2), 581–590. https://doi.org/10.1016/j.neuropsychologia.2009.10.021

Binder, L. M., Iverson, G. L., & Brooks, B. L. (2009). To err is human: "Abnormal" neuropsychological scores and variability are common in healthy adults. *Archives of Clinical Neuropsychology, 24*(1), 31–46. https://doi.org/10.1093/arclin/acn001

Chen, K.-L., Sun, Y.-M., Zhou, Y., Zhao, Q.-H., Ding, D., & Guo, Q.-H. (2016). Associations between APOE polymorphisms and seven diseases with cognitive impairment including Alzheimer's disease, frontotemporal dementia, and dementia with Lewy bodies in southeast China. *Psychiatric Genetics, 26*(3), 124–131. https://doi.org/10.1097/YPG.0000000000000126

Creswell, J. W., & Poth, C. N. (2017). *Qualitative Inquiry and Research Design. Choosing*

Among Five Approaches. Thousand Oaks, CA, USA: SAGE.

Delis, D. C., Kramer, J. H., Kaplan, E., & Ober, B. A. (2000). *California Verbal Learning Test, Second Edition*. San Antonio, TX, USA: Pearson.

Donovan, N. J., Wu, Q., Rentz, D. M., Sperling, R. A., Marshall, G. A., & Glymour, M. M. (2017). Loneliness, depression and cognitive function in older U.S. adults. *International Journal of Geriatric Psychiatry, 32*(5), 564–573. https://doi.org/10.1002/gps.4495

Edmonds, E. C., Delano-Wood, L., Galasko, D. R., Salmon, D. P., & Bondi, M. W. (2015). Subtle cognitive decline and biomarker staging in preclinical Alzheimer's disease. *Journal of Alzheimer's Disease, 47*(1), 231–242. https://doi.org/10.3233/JAD-150128

Farias, S. T., Mungas, D., Reed, B. R., Cahn-Weiner, D., Jagust, W., Baynes, K., & DeCarli, C. (2008). The Measurement of Everyday Cognition (ECog): Scale development and psychometric properties. *Neuropsychology, 22*(4), 531–544. https://doi.org/10.1037/0894-4105.22.4.531

Farrer, L. A., Cupples, A. L., Kukull, W. a, Mayeux, R., Myers, R. H., Pericak-vance, M. a, … van Duijn, C. M. (1997). Effects of age , sex , and ethnicity on the association between apolipoprotein E genotype and Alzheimer disease. *JAMA: The Journal of the American Medical Association, 278*, 1349–1356. https://doi.org/10.1001/jama.1997.03550160069041

Folstein, M. F., & Folstein, S. E. (2009). *Mini-Mental State Examination, 2nd edition*. Lutz, Fl, USA: PAR.

Gifford, K. A., Liu, D., Damon, S. M., Chapman, W. G., Romano, R. R., Samuels, L. R., … Jefferson, A. L. (2015). Subjective memory complaint only relates to verbal episodic memory performance in mild cognitive impairment. *Journal of Alzheimer's Disease, 44*(1), 309–318. https://doi.org/10.3233/JAD-140636

Graf, C. L. (2008). The Lawton Instrumental Activities of Daily Living Scale. *The American Journal of Nursing, 108*(4), 52-62.

Hokoishi, K., Ikeda, M., Maki, N., Nomura, M., Torikawa, S., Fujimoto, N., … Tanabe, H. (2001). Interrater reliability of the Physical Self-Maintenance Scale and the Instrumental Activities of Daily Living Scale in a variety of health professional representatives. *Aging and Mental Health, 5*(1), 38–40. https://doi.org/10.1080/13607860020020627

Hill, N. L., Mogle, J., Wion, R., Munoz, E., DePasquale, N., Yevchak, A. M., & Parisi, J. M. (2016). Subjective cognitive impairment and affective symptoms: A systematic review. *Gerontologist, 56*(6), e109–e127. https://doi.org/10.1093/geront/gnw091

Hsieh, H.-F., & Shannon, S. E. (2005). Three approaches to qualitative content analysis. *Qualitative Health Research, 15*(9), 1277–1288.

Ivnik, R. J., Malec, J. F., Smith, G. E., Tangalos, E. G., & Petersen, R. C. (1996). Neuropsychological tests' norms above age 55: COWAT, BNT, MAE token, WRAT-R reading, AMNART, STROOP, TMT, and JLO. *The Clinical Neuropsychologist, 10*(3), 262–278. https://doi.org/10.1080/13854049608406689

Jack, C. R., Bennett, D. A., Blennow, K., Carrillo, M. C., Dunn, B., Haeberlein, S. B., … Silverberg, N. (2018). NIA-AA Research Framework: Toward a biological definition of Alzheimer's disease. *Alzheimer's and Dementia, 14*(4), 535–562. https://doi.org/10.1016/j.jalz.2018.02.018

Jessen, F., Amariglio, R. E., Buckley, R. F., van der Flier, W. M., Han, Y., Molinuevo, J. L., … Wagner, M. (2020). The characterisation of subjective cognitive decline. *The Lancet Neurology, 19*(3), 271–278. https://doi.org/10.1016/S1474-4422(19)30368-0

Jessen, F., Amariglio, R. E., van Boxtel, M., Breteler, M., Ceccaldi, M., Chételat, G., …

Subjective Cognitive Decline Initiative (SCD-I) Working Group. (2014). A conceptual

framework for research on subjective cognitive decline in preclinical Alzheimer's disease.

Neuropsychology Review, *10*(6), 844–852. https://doi.org/10.1016/j.jalz.2014.01.001

Jiang, S., Tang, L., Zhao, N., Yang, W., Qiu, Y., & Chen, H. Z. (2016). A systems view of the

differences between APOE ε4 carriers and non-carriers in Alzheimer's disease. *Frontiers in*

Aging Neuroscience, *8*, 171. https://doi.org/10.3389/fnagi.2016.00171

Kaplan, E., Goodglass, H., & Weintraub, S. (2000). *Boston Naming Test, Second Edition*. San

Antonio, TX, USA: Pearson.

Krefting, L. (1991). Rigor in qualitative research: the assessment of trustworthiness. *The*

American Journal of Occupational Therapy. https://doi.org/10.5014/ajot.45.3.214

Kurt, P., Yener, G., & Oguz, M. (2011). Impaired digit span can predict further cognitive decline

in older people with subjective memory complaint: A preliminary result. *Aging & Mental*

Health, *15*(3), 364–369. https://doi.org/10.1080/13607863.2010.536133

Lezak, M. D., Howieson, D. B., Bigler, E. D., & Tranel, D. (2012). *Neuropsychological*

assessment, fifth edition. New York, NY, USA: Oxford University Press.

Lincoln, Y. S., & Guba, E. G. (1985). *Naturalistic inquiry*. Newbury Park, CA, USA: Sage.

Liu, Y., Tan, L., Wang, H.-F., Liu, Y., Hao, X.-K., Tan, C.-C., … Alzheimer's Disease

Neuroimaging Initiative. (2016). Multiple effect of APOE genotype on clinical and

neuroimaging biomarkers across Alzheimer's disease spectrum. *Molecular Neurobiology*,

53(7), 4539–4547. https://doi.org/10.1007/s12035-015-9388-7

Lowe, P. A., & Raad, J. M. (2006). Psychometric analyses of the AMAS-E scores in a sample of

older adults. *Individual Differences Research*, *4*(4), 272–290.

Lowe, P. A., & Reynolds, C. R. (2006). Examination of the psychometric properties of the Adult

Manifest Anxiety Scale-Elderly Version Scores. *Educational and Psychological*

Mast, B. T., & Gerstenecker, A. (2010). Screening instruments and brief batteries for dementia.

In P. A. Lichtenberg (Ed.), *Handbook of Assessment in Clinical Gerontology, Second*

Edition (pp. 503–530). Cambridge, MS, USA: Academic Press.

Mata, I. F., Leverenz, J. B., Weintraub, D., Trojanowski, J. Q., Hurtig, H. I., Van Deerlin, V. M.,

… Zabetian, C. P. (2014). APOE, MAPT, and SNCA genes and cognitive performance in

Parkinson disease. *JAMA Neurology, 71*(11), 1405–1412.

https://doi.org/10.1001/jamaneurol.2014.1455

Pink, A., Stokin, G. B., Bartley, M. M., Roberts, R. O., Sochor, O., Machulda, M. M., … Geda,

Y. E. (2015). Neuropsychiatric symptoms, APOE ε4, and the risk of incident dementia: A

population-based study. *Neurology, 84*(9), 935–943.

https://doi.org/10.1212/WNL.0000000000001307

Prestia, A., Caroli, A., Wade, S. K., van der Flier, W. M., Ossenkoppele, R., Van Berckel, B., …

Frisoni, G. B. (2015). Prediction of AD dementia by biomarkers following the NIA-AA and

IWG diagnostic criteria in MCI patients from three European memory clinics.

Neuropsychology Review, 11(10), 1191–1201. https://doi.org/10.1016/j.jalz.2014.12.001

Price, S. E., Kinsella, G. J., Ong, B., Storey, E., Mullaly, E., Phillips, M., … Perre, D. (2012).

Semantic verbal fluency strategies in amnestic mild cognitive impairment.

Neuropsychology, 26(4), 490–497. https://doi.org/10.1037/a0028567

Rabin, L. A., Borgos, M. J., Saykin, A. J., Wishart, H. A., Crane, P. K., Nutter-Upham, K. E., &

Flashman, L. A. (2007). Judgment in older adults: Development and psychometric

evaluation of the Test of Practical Judgment (TOP-J). *Journal of Clinical and Experimental*

Neuropsychology, 29(7), 752–767. https://doi.org/10.1080/13825580601025908

Rabin, L. A., Saykin, A. J., West, J. D., Borgos, M. J., Wishart, H. A., Nutter-Upham, K. E., …

Santulli, R. B. (2009). Judgment in older adults with normal cognition, cognitive

complaints, MCI, and mild AD: Relation to regional frontal gray matter. *Brain Imaging and

Behavior, 3*(2), 212–219. https://doi.org/10.1007/s11682-009-9063-6

Rabin, L. A., Saykin, A. J., Wishart, H. A., Nutter-Upham, K. E., Flashman, L. A., Pare, N., &

Santulli, R. B. (2007). The Memory and Aging Telephone Screen: Development and

preliminary validation. *Alzheimer's and Dementia, 3*(2), 109–121.

https://doi.org/10.1016/j.jalz.2007.02.002

Rabin, L. A., Smart, C. M., Crane, P. K., Amariglio, R. E., Berman, L. M., Boada, M., … Sikkes,

S. A. M. (2015). Subjective Cognitive Decline in Older Adults: An Overview of Self-

Report Measures Used Across 19 International Research Studies. *Journal of Alzheimer's

Disease : JAD, 48 Suppl 1*(s1), S63--86. https://doi.org/10.3233/JAD-150154

Rapp, M. A., & Reischies, F. M. (2005). Attention and executive control predict Alzheimer

disease in late life: Results from the Berlin Aging Study (BASE). *American Journal of

Geriatric Psychiatry, 13*(2), 134–141. https://doi.org/10.1097/00019442-200502000-00007

Rattanabannakit, C., Risacher, S. L., Gao, S., Lane, K. A., Brown, S. A., McDonald, B. C., …

Farlow, M. R. (2016). The Cognitive Change Index as a measure of self and informant

perception of cognitive decline: Relation to neuropsychological tests. *Journal of

Alzheimer's Disease, 51*(4), 1145–1155. https://doi.org/10.3233/JAD-150729

Reynolds, C. R., Richmond, B. O., Lowe, P. A. (2003). *Adult Manifest Anxiety Scale*. Torrance,

CA: Western Psychological Services.

Russell, D., Peplau, L. A., & Ferguson, M. L. (1978). Developing a measure of loneliness.

Journal of Personality Assessment, 42(3), 290–294.

https://doi.org/10.1207/s15327752jpa4203_11

Saykin, A. J., Wishart, H. A., Rabin, L. A., Santulli, R. B., Flashman, L. A., West, J. D., … Mamourian, A. C. (2006). Older adults with cognitive complaints show brain atrophy similar to that of amnestic MCI. *Neurology, 67*(5), 834–842.

Tandetnik, C., Hergueta, T., Bonnet, P., Dubois, B., & Bungener, C. (2017). Influence of early maladaptive schemas, depression, and anxiety on the intensity of self-reported cognitive complaint in older adults with subjective cognitive decline. *International Psychogeriatrics, 29*(10), 1657–1667.

Tomita, T., Sugawara, N., Kaneda, A., Okubo, N., Iwane, K., Takahashi, I., … Yasui-Furukori, N. (2014). Sex-specific effects of subjective memory complaints with respect to cognitive impairment or depressive symptoms. *Psychiatry and Clinical Neurosciences, 68*(3), 176–181. https://doi.org/10.1111/pcn.12102

Weakley, A., Schmitter-Edgecombe, M., & Anderson, J. (2013). Analysis of verbal fluency ability in amnestic and non-amnestic mild cognitive impairment. *Archives of Clinical Neuropsychology, 28*(7), 721–731. https://doi.org/10.1093/arclin/act058

Wechsler, D. (2008). *Wechsler Advanced Clinical Solutions for the WAIS-IV and WMS-IV*. San Antonio, TX, USA: Pearson.

Wechsler, D., & Psychological Corporation. (2008). *Wechsler Memory Scale, Fourth Edition*. San Antonio, TX, USA: The Psychological Corporation.

Weintraub, S., Besser, L., Dodge, H. H., Teylan, M., Ferris, S., Goldstein, F. C., … Morris, J. C. (2018). Version 3 of the Alzheimer Disease Centers' neuropsychological test battery in the Uniform Data Set (UDS). *Alzheimer Disease and Associated Disorders, 32*(1), 10–17. https://doi.org/10.1097/WAD.0000000000000223

Yesavage, J. A., Brink, T. L., Rose, T. L., Lum, O., Huang, V., Adey, M., & Leirer, V. O. (1982). Development and validation of a geriatric depression screening scale: A preliminary report. *Journal of Psychiatric Research, 17*(1), 1982–1983. https://doi.org/10.1016/0022-3956(82)90033-4

Appendix A: Consent Forms

Verbal Consent Script

Name: _______________________________

Telephone Number: _______________

Home Address: ____

Screening Date: ____

Hello,

I am returning your call about the Experiences with Aging study. Thank you for your interest. Your answers to this phone screen will help us determine whether or not you meet the eligibility requirements.

Is now still a good time for us to do the phone screen?   **Y**   N

You may discontinue this phone screen at any time for any reason.

Before we begin, I would like to tell you how we will handle the information you provide us in this phone screen. If, based on this information, you meet our initial eligibility criteria and you decide you would like to participate, this information will be part of your research file. This will be kept confidential and your name or other identifying information will be kept separate from your actual responses. If, however, based on this screen we determine that you are not eligible, we would still like to keep your information, but we will immediately remove all personally identifying information and make the data completely anonymous. The reason we would still want to keep the data even if you don't enroll in the study is so we may create statistics about how many interested people did and did not enroll.

Are you comfortable with us keeping your completely de-identified and anonymous information if you are not eligible for the study?   **Y**   **N**

Before we go on, let me ask you if you have any questions? If you are comfortable, do I have your permission to proceed?   **Y**   N

At this point, I would like to ask you some general background questions. You may stop at any time if you decide you are not comfortable.

***

Thank you. As you may remember, we are interested in the experience of older adults, particularly in areas of thinking and functioning that may or may not have changed over time. The purpose of this research is to learn more about these age-related experiences.

If you are found to be eligible, and if you are interested in participating, your participation will occur at the University of Victoria on two days of your choosing. You will be asked to come to our lab in the Psychology department with someone who knows you well (either a friend or a family member). After providing informed consent to participate in the study, you and your friend or family member will complete several short questionnaires about your moods and mental abilities. Your responses will be kept confidential and private from one another. Following this, you will participate in a cognitive assessment.

On another day, you will be invited to participate in a 1-hour interview with myself about your experiences with possible age-related changes. After this interview, you will be asked to spit into a tube so we may perform genetic testing. This sample will be used to test for potential markers of normal and non-normative cognitive changes. Given that your data will be anonymized, that genetic samples will be processed in batches, and that we have an incomplete knowledge of whether or which genetic markers may suggest potential for problems, we will not be able to share your specific genetic test results with you. That said, once this study is complete, we would be happy to share our overall results with you.

All together, we estimate your first visit should take 2 – 3 hours for you and about a half hour for your friend or family member. Your second visit should take no more than an hour and a half.

Before I proceed further, do you have any questions about this? Would this be agreeable to you?   **Y**   N

If you are comfortable, do I have your permission to proceed to our screening questions?   **Y**   N

UVic Experiences with Aging Study – Study Participant

This study will be conducted by Jordan I. Ali, MSc, principal investigator. Mr. Ali is a graduate student in the Department of Psychology at the University of Victoria. He is conducting this research as part of the requirements for his Doctoral degree in Clinical Neuropsychology.

This research is being conducted under the supervision of Dr. Colette Smart, registered psychologist and professor of Psychology at the University of Victoria. The Human Research Ethics Boards at the University of Victoria have approved the ethical conduct of this study.

What is the purpose of this study?
The goals of this study are to better understand how thinking abilities change with age. We would like to learn about your specific perceptions of and experiences with aging. The results of this study will be analyzed to determine whether there are any reliable differences between the experiences of those at lower and potentially higher risk of cognitive decline in late age.

If I choose to take part in this study, what will I do?
If you take part in this study, you will be invited to:

- Complete several questionnaires.
    You and a close friend/family member of your choosing will meet Mr. Ali at the University of Victoria campus to complete several questionnaires. Including the perspectives of close friends or family members is standard practice in this type of research and provides valuable information.

- Undergo a cognitive assessment.

You will take part in a comprehensive assessment of your
various thinking abilities. This testing is completely non-
invasive. This testing is expected to take approximately 2 hours.

- Participate in an interview about aging.
    You will speak with Mr. Ali for approximately 1 hour about
    your experiences with aging and potential changes in your
    thinking. Audio recordings and notes will be taken for the
    purpose of analysis and transcription.

- Provide a saliva sample.
    You will be asked to spit into a tube, which will then be sealed
    and sent to a lab for processing. We will be processing saliva
    samples in batches to determine the overall genetic profile of
    our study participants.

How long will this take?

Data collection will be split across two days of your choosing. The first day
will be dedicated to complete questionnaires and cognitive testing. This
day is expected to take up to 3 hours. The second day will be dedicated to
our interview and saliva sample collection. It is expected that this day will
take no longer than 1.5 hours.

Where will this take place?

This study will take place at the University of Victoria campus. Participants
will be asked to meet Mr. Ali in Cornett Building, Room A137.

Are there any risks or benefits associated with taking part in this study?

Risks: If you take part in this study, there is some chance that you may
experience some discomfort as a result of discussing potentially sensitive
or personal topics. In the event that this becomes overly distressing, you
may discontinue without any negative consequences. If this continues to
cause undue stress, Mr. Ali will consult with his supervisor, Dr. Smart, a
registered psychologist, to determine the appropriate course of action. If it

is appropriate that you receive follow-up counselling, we will provide you with a referral to the University of Victoria Psychology Clinic or another low-cost referral in the community.

Benefits: On the other hand, engaging with potentially sensitive or challenging topics may also help you come to terms with unresolved issues and/or gain a more positive perspective on your experiences. An additional benefit is that you will be contributing to our understanding of cognitive aging. It is possible that the information you and other study participants provide may help contribute to more effective support for older adults and more efficient identification of those at risk for cognitive issues in later life.

Will I receive any payment for taking part in the study?
You will be provided a $10 honorarium for each in-person session in acknowledgment and appreciation for your time.

During the study:
- You will be asked questions about your experiences and expectations of aging and potential age-related changes in thinking.

- You do not have to complete any tests that cause you undue discomfort, fatigue, or distress.

- The interview will be audio recorded for analysis and transcription.

- All information collected, including any possible identifying information, will be kept strictly confidential. However, if you disclose an intent to harm yourself or another, or child abuse at any time, we may be ethically and legally required to breach this confidentiality. If such a disclosure is made, Dr. Smart will be consulted and, if deemed necessary, the appropriate authorities will be informed.

- You may change your mind and withdraw from this study at any time. There is no need to explain why you have changed you mind.

- If you are not eligible or if you choose to withdraw from the study, we would still like to use any data already collected in our analysis. This data will help us describe the participants in the study. These data will be anonymous.

  Please check the box below and sign if you are comfortable with your anonymous data being used in the event of your withdrawal:

  ☐ Signature:____

After the study:
- Mr. Ali, Dr. Colette Smart, and research assistant(s) working on this study under our supervision will know that you have taken part on this study. They will be the only people who will have access to the information you shared unless otherwise indicated.

- Your name will not be recorded on the transcripts of your interview, your questionnaires, or your test results.

- Findings from this study will be reported in academic journals, Mr. Ali's Doctoral book (which may be published online), and presented at workshops/conferences. Your name will not be used in these publications or presentations.

- You will be contacted upon completion of the study and provided access to the study results and the resulting journal article(s) if you so wish.

- If you choose to withdraw, your decision to withdraw from the study will not affect your access to medical care or treatment.

- Information collected during the study will be stored in a locked filing cabinet in Dr. Smart's lab space and on an encrypted and password-protected hard drive for 7 years. At the end of this time, all paper records will be shredded and all audiotapes will be deleted.

- In addition to the current study, you may be eligible for other aging studies being conducted at the University of Victoria.

  Please check the box below and sign if you would like to be contacted to participate in additional aging studies at the University of Victoria:

  ☐ Signature:____

  If you are interested in participating in additional studies, it may be helpful for us to share your data openly with the other researchers you are involved with. If this was to occur, your confidentiality would be maintained outside the specific studies you have participated in.

  Please check the box below and sign if you would be comfortable with your data from this study being openly shared with any other researchers you are involved with:

  ☐ Signature:____

- It is possible that a follow-up study will be conducted in the future. We would like to retain your contact information for up to 10 years so that, if a follow-up study is undertaken, you will be contacted and given the option to participate.

  Please check the box below and sign if you are comfortable with your contact information being retained for 10 years in case of a possible follow up study:

☐ Signature:____

**If you have any questions or if you would like to discuss this study
further, please contact Jordan I. Ali, MSc.**
>   **Phone: 250-472-4194   e-mail: jali@uvic.ca**

If you have any questions you would like to direct to the faculty
supervisor, please contact Dr. Colette Smart.
>   Phone: 250-853-3997   e-mail: csmart@uvic.ca

The Human Research Ethics Boards at the University of Victoria have
approved the ethical conduct of this research.

If you have any questions regarding the ethical conduct of this research,
please contact the Human Research Ethics Office.
>   Phone: 250-472-4545   e-mail: ethics@uvic.ca.

Please remember that your participation in this study is voluntary

Consent:

I have read this consent letter   Initial______

I have had the opportunity to ask questions   Initial______

I understand that my participation in this study is voluntary   Initial______

I understand that I can withdraw my consent at any time   Initial______

I understand that my interview will be audio taped   Initial______

I agree to take part in the study   Initial______

Name of Participant: ____

Signature: ____

Date: ____

Telephone: ____

Email: ____

Witness: ____

Date: ____

A copy of this consent letter will be left with you, and the researcher will take a copy.

Appendix B: Questionnaires

Revised Memory and Aging Telephone Screen (Rabin et al., 2007)

DEMOGRAPHICS

Date of Birth: _____________   Age: __

Sex: M   F   other

Handedness: R   L   ambi

Highest Level of Educational Achievement (e.g., grade X, diploma, BA, PhD, etc.):   __

Are you retired?   Y   N   What is/was your profession: _____________________

English as first language?   Y   N
    If no: At what age did you learn English? _______
    If no: What is the primary language spoken at home? _______________
    If no: Are you fluent in English speech?   **Y**   N
    If no: Are you fluent in English reading/writing?   **Y**   N

Do you have normal or corrected-to-normal vision?   **Y**   N
Do you have double vision?   Y   **N**
Are you colour blind?   Y   **N**

Do you have any hearing impairment?   Y   N
    If yes: do you use a hearing aid?   Y   N

Have you had any major medical problems or surgeries? _____________________________

Have you ever been diagnosed with a neurological disease, such as stroke or epilepsy?
    Y   **N**
    If yes: Please explain: _______________________________________

Have you ever been diagnosed with a memory problem or dementia? Y   **N**
    If yes: What was the diagnosis? _______________________________

Have you ever been diagnosed with a traumatic brain injury (not including concussion)?
    Y   **N**
    If yes: Please explain: _______________________________________

Have you ever had a concussion?   Y   N
    If yes: When did you experience this concussion? _______
    If yes: Did you lose consciousness as a result of this concussion?   Y   N
        If yes: For how long? _______ hours
    If yes: Was the concussion diagnosed by a professional (e.g., doctor, etc.)?   Y   N

COGNITIVE CONCERNS

I would like to ask you about your memory specifically. Do you have any difficulties with:

Problem Area	*Description/Details*	*circle one:*
1. Remembering conversations?		N Y DK
2. Word finding (e.g., coming up with the right word; tip-of-the-tongue)		N Y DK
3. Compared to your peers, do you think you have more difficulty remembering names?		N Y DK
4. Compared to your peers, do you think you have more difficulty learning new information?		N Y DK
5. Finding everyday objects? (e.g., wallets, keys)		N Y DK
6. Remembering what you entered a room to do?		N Y DK
7. How is your memory now compared to the best it's ever been?		Same Worse
8. Is it worse than for others your age?		N Y DK
9. Does it affect daily activities? (e.g., social, vocational, recreational)		N Y DK
10. How long ago/when did your memory problems start?	Age at onset: _______ Duration: __ yrs ___ mos	
11. Have they gotten worse over time?		N Y DK
12. Have you sought evaluation or treatment of your memory problems? (list tests & medications tried)	When?: ____	N Y DK
13. Any other problems with your memory?		N Y DK

** **Are these changes to your memory or any other thinking abilties concerning to you (e.g., more than you would expect compared to others your age)?**   Y   N

TRIAL 1:	I would like to get a preliminary sense of your memory ability. I will read a list of words to you and have you repeat back as many words as you can in any order. *(Read one word per second, clearly and slowly)*
TRIALS 2, 3:	That was good. I would like you to do the same thing again. I am going to read the list and I would like you to tell me back as many words as you can, in any order, including ones from the list you've already said.

LIST	TRIAL 1	TRIAL 2	TRIAL 3
hat	1.	1.	1.
engine	2.	2.	2.
dancer	3.	3.	3.
fort	4.	4.	4.
chair	5.	5.	5.
garden	6.	6.	6.
apron	7.	7.	7.
crystal	8.	8.	8.
face	9.	9.	9.
pill	10.	10.	10.
	11.	11.	11.
	12.	12.	12.
	13.	13.	13.
	14.	14.	14.
	15.	15.	15.

Time complete: __:___

Note: There should be a 10 – 20 minute delay to delayed free recall.

****

If you think you may like to participate in this study, I'd like to ask you some more questions regarding factors we need to evaluate for your eligibility.

***

PHYSICAL HEALTH

Name of physician: ______________________________________

Do you have hypertension/high blood pressure?   Y   N
      If yes: Are you on medication to control hypertension?   Y   N
      If yes: Is it well-controlled?:   Y   N

Do you have high cholesterol?   Y   N
      If yes: Do you take medication to control your cholesterol?   Y   N

Are you taking medications?   Y   N
      If yes:

Medication	Purpose

Have you ever had cancer?   Y   N
      If yes: what type? ______________________________
      If yes: Have you ever undergone radiation?   Y   N
      If yes: Have you ever undergone chemotherapy?   Y   N

Have you ever had heart problems?   Y   N
      If yes: Please explain: __________________________________

Do you have problems regulating your blood sugar?   Y   N
      If yes: Please explain: _______________________________

Do you have any other (physical) health issues?   Y   N
      If yes: Please explain: _____________________

____

How much do you sleep on average? __ hours

Do you have any issues with sleep (e.g., insomnia, apnea)?   Y   N
      If yes: Please explain: ___________________________

Any changes in your sleep recently?   Y   N

If yes: Please explain: _______________________________

Any changes in your appetite recently?   Y   N
        If yes: Please explain: ____

How often do you drink alcohol?   _______________
        How much alcohol do you drink on these occasions? _______________

Do you smoke cigarettes or otherwise use tobacco?   Y   N
        If yes: how many cigarettes do you smoke per day? _________/day

Do you wear a nicotine patch? Y   N

Do you use marijuana or marijuana products? Y   N
        If yes: How often do you use marijuana or marijuana products? _______
        If yes: Is your marijuana prescribed?   Y   N

Do you use any other non-prescribed substances?   Y   N
        If yes: Please explain: ____

MENTAL/COGNITIVE HEALTH

Has anyone in your family ever been diagnosed with a memory problem or dementia?
        Y   N
        If yes: What was the diagnosis? _________________________________
        If yes: Was this person a first-degree relative (e.g., parent, sibling, child)?
        Y   N

How concerned are you about the possibility of developing dementia?

0 = Not at all concerned	1 = Slightly concerned	2 = Somewhat concerned	3 = Quite concerned	4 = Very concerned

Have you ever been diagnosed with a psychological condition (e.g., including depression, anxiety)?
        Y   N
        If yes: What was the diagnosis? _________________________________

Have you ever had severe headaches or migraines?   Y   N

<table>
<tr><td>**DELAYED RECALL**</td><td>A little while ago, I read a list of words to you. I would like you to tell me as many of those words as you can recall now.</td></tr>
<tr><td>**RECOGNITION**</td><td>I am now going to read some more words to you. I want you to tell me "yes" if the word was on the list I read to you, and "no" if the word was not on the list I read to you.</td></tr>
</table>

DELAYED RECALL

RECOGNITION

DELAYED RECALL						
1.	**apron**	Y	N	target	Y	**N**
2.	mud	Y	**N**	heart	Y	**N**
3.	captain	Y	**N**	person	Y	**N**
4.	**dancer**	Y	N	feather	Y	**N**
5.	**pill**	**Y**	N	cigar	Y	**N**
6.	food	Y	**N**	angel	Y	**N**
7.	pansy	Y	**N**	cat	Y	**N**
8.	door	Y	**N**	hotel	Y	**N**
9.	tower	Y	**N**	**engine**	**Y**	N
10.	**face**	**Y**	N	stomach	Y	**N**
11.	paste	Y	**N**	ring	Y	**N**
12.	**chair**	**Y**	N	cellar	Y	**N**
13.	budget	Y	**N**	**crystal**	**Y**	N
14.	park	Y	**N**	**garden**	**Y**	N
15.	dress	Y	**N**	parade	Y	**N**
	smile	Y	**N**	tiger	Y	**N**
	pocket	Y	**N**	**hat**	**Y**	N
	seed	Y	**N**	dairy	Y	**N**
	leg	Y	**N**	spot	Y	**N**
	fort	**Y**	N	ocean	Y	**N**

GENETIC TESTING

Have you ever done any direct-to-consumer genetic testing (e.g., 23andMe, Ancestry.com)?
    Y   N

    If yes: Were you given your APOE genotype?   Y   N
        If yes: What was it? ______________________________

INFORMANT

Do you have a person who knows you well and with whom you have at least 6 hours per week of direct or phone contact, and who could answer questions about your memory and general health?   **Y**   N

    Name: ____

    Relationship: ____

SOURCE

How did you hear about this study?   ______________________________

What was the *main* factor leading you to volunteer?:

    A. I am concerned about my memory or other thinking abilities
        Please explain (e.g., due to family Hx, observed changes, etc.):
        ____
        ____

    B. I am interested in helping with research
    C. Other
        Please explain: ______________________________

The Lawton Instrumental Activities of Daily Living Scale

A. Ability to Use Telephone
1. Operates telephone on own initiative; looks up and dials numbers............ 1
2. Dials a few well-known numbers............ 1
3. Answers telephone, but does not dial............ 1
4. Does not use telephone at all............ 0

B. Shopping
1. Takes care of all shopping needs independently............ 1
2. Shops independently for small purchases............ 0
3. Needs to be accompanied on any shopping trip............ 0
4. Completely unable to shop............ 0

C. Food Preparation
1. Plans, prepares, and serves adequate meals independently............ 1
2. Prepares adequate meals if supplied with ingredients............ 0
3. Heats and serves prepared meals or prepares meals but does not maintain adequate diet............ 0
4. Needs to have meals prepared and served............ 0

D. Housekeeping
1. Maintains house alone with occasion assistance (heavy work)............ 1
2. Performs light daily tasks such as dishwashing, bed making............ 1
3. Performs light daily tasks, but cannot maintain acceptable level of cleanliness............ 1
4. Needs help with all home maintenance tasks............ 1
5. Does not participate in any housekeeping tasks............ 0

E. Laundry
1. Does personal laundry completely............ 1
2. Launders small items, rinses socks, stockings, etc............ 1
3. All laundry must be done by others............ 0

F. Mode of Transportation
1. Travels independently on public transportation or drives own car............ 1
2. Arranges own travel via taxi, but does not otherwise use public transportation............ 1
3. Travels on public transportation when assisted or accompanied by another............ 1
4. Travel limited to taxi or automobile with assistance of another............ 0
5. Does not travel at all............ 0

G. Responsibility for Own Medications
1. Is responsible for taking medication in correct dosages at correct time............ 1
2. Takes responsibility if medication is prepared in advance in separate dosages............ 0
3. Is not capable of dispensing own medication............ 0

H. Ability to Handle Finances
1. Manages financial matters independently (budgets, writes checks, pays rent and bills, goes to bank); collects and keeps track of income............ 1
2. Manages day-to-day purchases, but needs help with banking, major purchases, etc............ 1
3. Incapable of handling money............ 0

Scoring: For each category, circle the item description that most closely resembles the client's highest functional level (either 0 or 1).

Lawton, M.P., & Brody, E.M. (1969). Assessment of older people: Self-maintaining and instrumental activities of daily living. *The Gerontologist, 9*(3), 179-186.

Key Item	Possible Queries (phrasing may vary)
Tell me about your **thinking abilities** as you have gotten older?	(Q) In the past 5 years or so? (Q) What, if anything, has gotten more challenging for you? (Q) What, if anything, has gotten easier for you? (Q) What, if anything, has stayed the same for you?
How has your **processing speed** been (e.g., the speed with which you are able to think and process information)? *Provide examples as necessary*	(Q) What has changed (as you have gotten older/in the past 5 years)? (Q) What is just as it has always been? (Q) How about your ability to keep up with conversations? (Q) How about your ability to notice and respond to things? (Q) Has that gotten in the way of your doing the things you would like to/are used to doing? …How has that gotten in the way/what has that gotten in the way of? (Q) What do you do to help yourself keep up (better)?
How has your **attention** been? *Provide examples as necessary*	(Q) What has changed (as you have gotten older/in the past 5 years)? (Q) What is just as it has always been? (Q) How about your ability to focus on things? (Q) How about your ability to concentrate for longer periods of time? (Q) Do you feel you are more distractible? …By external stimuli (e.g., sounds, etc.)? …By internal stimuli (e.g., preoccupied by worries, etc.)? (Q) Do you find paying attention takes more effort than before? (Q) Has that gotten in the way of your doing the things you would like to/are used to doing? …How has that gotten in the way/what has that gotten in the way of? (Q) What do you do to help yourself pay attention more (easily)?

Key Item	Possible Queries (phrasing may vary)
How has your **working memory** been (e.g., your ability to keep information in mind for a time)? *Provide examples as necessary*	(Q) What has changed (as you have gotten older/in the past 5 years)? (Q) What is just as it has always been? (Q) How about your ability to keep information in mind for a short time? (Q) How about your ability to keep track of what you were doing? (Q) Has that gotten in the way of your doing the things you would like to/are used to doing? …How has that gotten in the way/what has that gotten in the way of? (Q) What do you do to help yourself keep information in mind (better)?
How has your **memory** been (e.g., learning and recall)? *Provide examples as necessary*	(Q) What has changed (as you have gotten older/in the past 5 years)? (Q) What is just as it has always been? (Q) How about your ability to learn new information? (Q) Do you find learning takes more effort than before? (Q) How about your ability remember things? …Events from the distant past? …Events from the recent past? …Information that you know/once knew well? …Names? …Activities? (Q) How about your ability to remember dates and appointments? (Q) How about your ability to remember to do things later? (Q) Has that gotten in the way of your doing the things you would like to/are used to doing? …How has that gotten in the way/what has that gotten in the way of? (Q) What do you do to help yourself learn/remember more (easily)?

Key Item	Possible Queries (phrasing may vary)
How has your **language** been (e.g., your ability to understand and communicate)? *Provide examples as necessary*	(Q) What has changed (as you have gotten older/in the past 5 years)? (Q) What is just as it has always been? (Q) How about your ability to understand when people are speaking to you? …How about if your hearing was 100%. How would it be, then? (Q) How about your ability to communicate clearly? …Has there been any change in your ability to stay on topic? …Has there been any change in how direct you are in your speech? (Q) How about your ability to find the right word at the right time? (Q) Has that gotten in the way of your doing the things you would like to/are used to doing? …How has that gotten in the way/what has that gotten in the way of? (Q) What do you do to help yourself understand/communicate (more clearly)?
How has your **visuospatial functioning** been (e.g., navigation/orientation)? *Provide examples as necessary*	(Q) What has changed (as you have gotten older/in the past 5 years)? (Q) What is just as it has always been? (Q) How about your ability to find your way to/in familiar locations? (Q) How about your ability to find your way back when you get turned around/lost? (Q) Has that gotten in the way of your doing the things you would like to/are used to doing? …How has that gotten in the way/what has that gotten in the way of? (Q) What do you do to help yourself navigate?

Key Item	Possible Queries (phrasing may vary)
How has your **executive functioning** been (e.g., multitasking, problem-solving)? *Provide examples as necessary*	(Q) What has changed (as you have gotten older/in the past 5 years)? (Q) What is just as it has always been? (Q) How about your ability to multitask? …How about doing several things at the same time? …How about switching back and forth between tasks? (Q) How about your ability to problem-solve? (Q) How about your ability to make (good) decisions? (Q) Have you become more impulsive over time? (Q) Have you noticed difficulties "switching gears"? (Q) Have you noticed difficulties with planning or carrying out activities in a specific sequence? (Q) Has that gotten in the way of your doing the things you would like to/are used to doing? …How has that gotten in the way/what has that gotten in the way of? (Q) What do you do to help yourself multitask/stay on top of things (better)?
How has your **mood** been? *Provide examples as necessary*	(Q) What has changed (as you have gotten older/in the past 5 years)? (Q) What is just as it has always been? (Q) Has your mood declined more/been lower? (Q) Have you felt more anxious? …Do you find it difficult to turn off your worries? …Do you feel overwhelmed? (Q) Has that gotten in the way of your doing the things you would like to/are used to doing? …How has that gotten in the way/what has that gotten in the way of? (Q) What do you do to help yourself navigate?

Key Item	Possible Queries (phrasing may vary)
How often does that happen for you? (for all reported areas of change)	(Q) Is that a change from before? (Q) How do you feel about that?
Does that cause you any **concern**? (for all reported areas of change) *Differentiate concern from change or functional disruption as necessary*	(Q) How do you feel about that? (Q) Do those changes make you worried? …What are you worried about? (Q) Do you think these changes are pathological? …What do you think might be happening? …Do you think these are expected changes for older adults?

Appendix D: Debriefing Script

The purpose of the study you just completed was to investigate the specific nature of perceived cognitive changes and concerns about cognitive change among people with varying levels of risk for objective cognitive decline. Research shows that for some people, cognitive concerns may be a sign of underlying pathology; however, we currently know very little about when or for whom this is the case. The information you provided will help us gain a better understanding of what age-related concerns may or may not be typical for older adults.

As we discussed at the beginning of this study, although we will be performing genetic testing, we will not be able to provide you with your personal results. We will be analyzing all of our genetic information in batches and will have difficulty determining whose specific samples are connected to specific datasets. Additionally, since it remains unclear how predictive certain genetic markers are of any pathology, we cannot be certain of the meaning of any genetic results in isolation.

Your data will also be compared to others like you to determine which changes/concerns are most common among older adults and which may be more atypical. Our hope is that all of this information may allow us to create clinical measures to better identify when people are at risk for developing cognitive issues.

If you have indicated interest in participating in additional studies, your name will be forwarded to the other members of the research team and you will be contacted shortly to discuss further research opportunities.

It will likely be some time until this project is completed and the data analyzed, but we would be happy to follow up with you once we have the overall results worked out. Would you be interested in that? We thank you for your participation.

Chapter 3: Parsing the predictive potential of subjective cognitive decline and subtle cognitive decline for dementia risk.

Introduction

Subjective cognitive decline (SCD) has been defined as a self-perceived decline in cognitive function among older adults in spite of performing within normal limits on standardized clinical-neuropsychological tests (Jessen et al., 2014). In recent years, SCD has attracted a great deal of attention as a potential prodrome of Alzheimer's disease (AD) and other forms of objective late-life cognitive dysfunction, such as mild cognitive impairment (MCI). While concerns regarding cognition may not be entirely rare among older adults (Cooper et al., 2011; Jonker, Geerlings, & Schmand, 2000), there is persuasive evidence to suggest that, for at least a subset of those with SCD, self-perceived changes in cognitive functioning may indeed herald eventual decline to dementia (Reisberg, Shulman, Torossian, Leng, & Zhu, 2010). Supporting this, numerous studies have found an association between the presence of SCD and AD-consistent pathological markers, including hippocampal atrophy (Cherbuin, Sargent-Cox, Easteal, Sachdev, & Anstey, 2015), amyloid deposition (Amariglio et al., 2012), and volumetric change in cerebrospinal fluid (Robert Stewart et al., 2011). The relationship between SCD and cognitive dysfunction may be stronger still where persons with SCD carry the APOE ε4 gene, an oft-cited risk factor for pathological cognitive decline (Ali, Smart, & Gawryluk, 2018).

Combined, this evidence suggests that SCD may not only represent the earliest preclinical form of AD and other neurodegenerative processes, but also an ideal window for intervention before objective impairment manifests (Imtiaz, Tolppanen, Kivipelto, & Soininen, 2014; Smart et al., 2017). At the least, it has been argued that the mere presence of SCD may serve as a screening tool to identify those at-risk of dementia who may be most amenable to preventative efforts (Buckley et al., 2016; Lista et al., 2015). Unfortunately, due to a lack of reliable and accurate means to identify high-risk individuals with SCD, this clinical potential has yet to be realized.

Challenges to Isolating SCD-Related Risk

Multi-determination. A core challenge with distinguishing age-normative concerns from potentially pathological concerns associated with SCD is the multi-determined nature of SCD. While it is true that SCD has been linked to underlying neuropathological processes (Ali et al., 2018), it has also been shown that SCD is highly correlated with psychological factors, such as trait neuroticism, anxiety, and depression (Comijs, Deeg, Dik, Twisk, & Jonker, 2002; Derouesné, Lacomblez, Thibault, & LePoncin, 1999; Dux et al., 2008; Jenkins, Tree, Thornton, & Tales, 2019; Slavin et al., 2010). These factors may, in turn, be influenced by other situational factors and medical comorbidities, such as chronic pain, which is relatively common in older adults (Allaz & Cedraschi, 2015; Gibson, 2015; Goesling, Clauw, & Hassett, 2013). Given that SCD may result from multiple etiologies, and that not all of these relate to risk of AD or other dementias, it has proven difficult to distinguish SCD that is potentially prodromal to a dementia process from SCD due to other factors (Tuokko & Smart, 2018).

Insensitive measures. Individuals with SCD perform within normal limits on objective cognitive tests by definition (Jessen et al., 2014). Nevertheless, numerous attempts have been made to identify SCD-specific cognitive profiles that are indicative of underlying neuropathology. These attempts have met with limited success. Individuals with SCD have occasionally been found to perform more poorly than healthy controls (without SCD) on cognitive screening measures (Stewart et al., 2001), as well as clinical tests of simple attention (Fortea et al., 2011), memory (Jessen et al., 2007), and executive functioning (Fonseca et al., 2015); however, these results have not been consistently replicated. This mixed outcome is not entirely unexpected given the psychometric properties of standardized clinical-neuropsychological measures, which aim to detect cognitive impairment significant enough to impact daily functioning. In service of this goal, clinical impairment thresholds are conservative by design to optimize diagnostic sensitivity. The result is that such tests perform well in identifying those with frank impairment but are relatively insensitive to incremental differences in normal-range, unimpaired performance. While such measures have proven invaluable for identifying clinical samples, they are less well-equipped to assess subclinical decrements as may be present in SCD.

The Role of Biomarker Data in SCD Risk Assessment

The clinical significance and reliability of SCD risk assessment could be bolstered by the inclusion of known biological risk markers (e.g., biomarkers), as these provide objective data free from psychometric shortcomings or psychosocial influences. A prime candidate for this risk marker may be the APOE ε4 genotype. While many biomarkers are not easily accessible to clinicians outside major research centres (e.g., PiB-PET; Perrotin, Mormino, Madison, Hayenga, & Jagust, 2012), APOE ε4 genotype is easily obtained through low-cost non-invasive methods, and has shown promise in differentiating those with AD-predicting SCD from those with SCD associated with other etiologies (Krell-Roesch et al., 2015). Further, APOE ε4 has been consistently identified as a risk factor for conversion to AD and vascular dementia (Allan & Ebmeier, 2011; Chen et al., 2016; Jiang et al., 2016; Liu et al., 2016; Mata et al., 2014; Pink et al., 2015; Prestia et al., 2015). APOE ε4 carriers have been estimated to have approximately three times greater risk of developing AD, while double allele carriers are estimated to be approximately 15 times more likely than the general population to develop AD (Farrer et al., 1997). With respect to SCD, a recent review found that APOE ε4 does not impact the development of SCD (broadly defined), but that SCD and APOE ε4 confer independent and interacting risk for conversion to an objectively cognitively impaired state (Ali et al., 2018). Given the relationship between SCD, APOE ε4, and AD-consistent neuropathology, the APOE ε4 genotype may provide crucial insight into risk for cognitive decline among those with SCD and may contextualize otherwise ambiguous evidence provided through other approaches. It is for exactly this reason that both the SCD Plus guidelines for high-risk SCD (Jessen et al., 2014) and NIA preclinical AD criteria (Jack et al., 2018) encourage the collection of biomarker data to supplement neuropsychological test scores when assessing cognitive risk.

Subtle Cognitive Decline as a Potential Indicator of Incipient Cognitive Decline

Due to the aforementioned limitations, determining an at-risk cognitive profile or cognitive test performance threshold has proven challenging; nevertheless, the construct of subtle cognitive decline (subtle CD) may yet provide a means to derive risk for pathological decline from objective quantitative data. In 2011, the National Institute on Aging and the Alzheimer's Association (NIA-AA) proposed research criteria for preclinical AD (Sperling et al., 2011). These criteria assumed a chronological development of AD risk factors, beginning with cerebral amyloid accumulation, then advancing to neurodegeneration, and culminating in subtle CD before the onset of frank dementia. However, while the risk biomarkers were concretely defined and allowed for additional investigation, subtle CD was not described further. Although subtle CD was considered the behavioural manifestation of well-developed neurological vulnerabilities, the construct added little to the preclinical AD literature when left purely as a qualitative label. Thus, in order to include it in their investigation of the validity of the NIA-AA's criteria for preclinical AD, Edmonds and colleagues undertook to operationalize subtle CD more concretely (Edmonds, Delano-Wood, Galasko, Salmon, & Bondi, 2015).

Upon follow-up, a number of Edmonds et al.'s healthy adult sample had developed objective cognitive impairment. Of those who presented with only one NIA-AA risk factor at baseline, subtle CD was just as likely to present as amyloidosis. Subtle CD was included in 8% of converted cases where two risk factors were identified at baseline. Further, of those presenting with all three of amyloidosis, neurodegeneration, and subtle CD at baseline, approximately 24% developed eventual objective cognitive impairment. Having any two or more risk factors was associated with a significantly increased risk of developing objective cognitive impairment. Considering the NIA-AA's stipulation that subtle CD may be the final manifestation of underlying pathology before the onset of frank impairment, the increased risk posed by subtle CD when paired with other risk factors, and its amenability to non-invasive and economical screening, subtle CD may present a powerful indicator of potential cognitive risk.

Research Objectives

Owing to the early and exploratory nature of this work, guiding research objectives were established in lieu of concrete hypotheses. Our overarching aim was to elucidate the relationship(s) between SCD, APOE ε4 genotype, specific psychosocial factors, and potential prodromal pathological cognitive decline. In service of this goal, our specific research objectives were duple. First, in light of the multi-determined nature of SCD, we aimed to 1) isolate the specific psychosocial, cognitive, and genetic factors that contribute most to SCD endorsement among older adult community samples. Next, we aimed to 2) clarify whether and to what extent SCD endorsement and APOE ε4 genotype relate to objective cognitive performance (i.e, subtle CD).

Methods

Participants

Eligible participants were adults >65 years of age living independently in British Columbia, Canada. In line with Jessen and coworkers' negative criteria of cognitive or functional impairment (Jessen et al., 2014), eligible participants had never received a diagnosis related to cognitive impairment or any specific neurological disorder (e.g., dementia, stroke, etc.) and were

138

cognitively and functionally intact. Potential participants were considered to have probable MCI and, consequently, were excluded from analyses if they a) achieved a *z*-score <2.00 on the Memory and Aging Telephone Screen (Rabin et al., 2007); b) achieved a score <24 on the MMSE-2 cognitive screening measure, c) achieved a score <8 on the Lawton-Brody IADL scale, or d) scored >1 standard deviation below the age-normative mean across the majority of neuropsychological tests loading onto any single cognitive domain (Edmonds et al., 2015). After screening, *n*=65 participants met eligibility criteria.

SCD determination. A substantial body of work has demonstrated that cognitive complaints and self-reported declines are typical of the aging experience and, as such, may provide limited benefit for predicting an individuals' cognitive trajectory. Conversely, it has been suggested that *concerns* about cognitive decline are significantly more predictive of later declines (Jessen et al., 2014). Thus, the classification of SCD endorsement in the current study was informed by Subjective Cognitive Decline Initiative (SCD-I) Working Group's criteria for SCD that is high risk for AD (SCD *Plus*; Jessen et al., 2014) and corroborating studies (Jessen et al., 2020; Jessen et al., 2014; Rabin et al., 2015). Participants' SCD endorsement was determined by first exploring whether they had noticed any cognitive changes/declines within the past five years and then following up with a single query: "Are your cognitive changes concerning to you (e.g., more than you would expect compared to others your age)?".

Subtle CD classification. In addition to the classification of SCD based on self-identification, participants were classified as healthy controls or as demonstrating subtle CD based on their neuropsychological test performance. We applied Edmonds and colleagues' criteria for subtle CD with few amendments to better suit the large battery used in this study (Edmonds et al., 2015). Specifically, Edmonds et al. administered an abbreviated battery of six tests divided equally across three cognitive domains (i.e., two tests per domain). Their criteria state that individuals with a single score >1 SD below age-normed mean distributed across each of two neuropsychological domains may be assumed to have declined from their previous/expected level of ability and, consequently, were considered to demonstrate subtle CD. In contrast, individuals with more than one low score within a domain or with a single low score in each of the three domains were considered to have probable MCI.

Previous work demonstrates the high probability – even typicality – of scores >1 SD below age-normed means even in healthy individuals (Binder, Iverson, & Brooks, 2009). Given the increased likelihood of familywise error due to the greater number of tests administered in the current study, we retained Edmonds et al.'s inclusion criteria for subtle CD but discarded their frequency-based criterion for exclusion (i.e., MCI) in favor of a percentage-based criterion (i.e., if >50% of an individual's scores within a given cognitive domain are >1 standard deviation below the age-normative mean, they are considered to have MCI and were ineligible for inclusion). We believe this amendment stays true to the intent of Edmonds et al.'s definition while allowing for its application to a more comprehensive battery.

Thus, participants were categorized as healthy controls (absent subtle CD) or as evidencing subtle CD. Each group was then further sub-divided according to the presence or absence of self-identified SCD as described above.

Measures and Materials

Self-report measures. Participants completed self-report scales related to depression, anxiety, and self-perceived cognitive and daily functioning.

Adult Manifest Anxiety Scale, elderly version (AMAS-E; Reynolds, Richmond, Lowe, 2003). The AMAS has been found to be temporally stable, to have moderate to good correlation with other established measures (Lowe & Raad, 2006), and to be invariant with gender (Lowe & Reynolds, 2006). All forms of the AMAS include a validity scale which may provide insight into participants' openness to endorsing symptoms. The AMAS-E specifically contains subscales dedicated to worry/oversensitivity, physiological anxiety, and fear of aging in adults 60 years of age and older. The inclusion of the AMAS-E was key in our investigation of SCD and subtle CD. Anxiety has been consistently linked to the endorsement of SCD (e.g., Hill et al., 2016; Tandetnik et al., 2017). The role of anxiety in subtle CD remains unclear. Including the AMAS-E general score and subscale score as predictors allowed us to determine the extent to which various dimensions of anxiety contributed to our constructs of interest.

Cognitive Change Index (CCI; Saykin et al., 2006). The CCI measures individuals' perceptions of cognitive change over time across several cognitive domains, including memory, language, and executive functioning. The CCI scores correspond relatively well with objective test performance (Rattanabannakit et al., 2016). High scores on the CCI indicate a greater degree of perceived cognitive change. Although the CCI's content clearly overlaps with perceived cognitive change, it is less clear whether it reflects the concern aspect of SCD. Further, it is unclear whether the CCI may be a good measure of objective cognitive changes in the earliest stages (as might be manifested by subtle CD). The CCI was included as a predictor in accordance with our overarching goal to identify potential screening measures and items that are particularly sensitive to risky conditions, like SCD and subtle CD.

Demographics and health history. A demographics and physical/mental health history questionnaire was created for use in this study. Questionnaire items queried general demographic details (e.g., age, sex, education, etc.), presence of physical health adversities known to impact cognitive functioning, previous and/or current mental health adversities, family history of cognitive disorder, and previous genetic testing experience. Age, sex, and education have each been found to impact the endorsement of SCD and, thus, were included as predictor variables. Advanced age is strongly associated with increased risk for pathological cognitive decline. Sex (and related socialization) has been found to exert an influence on who is likely to endorse cognitive concerns and at what stage of development or severity. Education, on the other hand, is a key contributor to cognitive reserve (e.g., resilience against pathological cognitive decline bestowed by one's education and socioeconomic standing), which has been shown to impact the alacrity and trajectory of cognitive decline once pathology has been established (e.g., Stern, 2012). Additionally, positive psychiatric history and family history of dementia/cognitive disorder were also included as predictors due to their demonstrated influence on dementia risk.

Geriatric Depression Scale, short form (GDS; Yesavage et al., 1982). The GDS is designed to reflect the unique presentation of depression in older adults, controlling for physical symptoms and health adversities. The GDS has been shown to have predictive validity in terms of quality of life, independent activities of daily living, and depressive mood, and has proven reliable with older adult populations (Cronbach's alpha .90). The GDS was included as a predictor given its frequent use for screening purposes and evidence that depressive symptoms may both speed cognitive decline (Kim et al., 2015; Müller-Gerards et al., 2019) and influence self-reported cognitive functioning and concern (Tomita et al., 2014).

Measurement of Everyday Cognition, select subscales (ECog; Farias et al., 2008). The full ECog measures self-reported cognitive ability relative to same-aged peers across six domains, including memory, language, visuospatial ability, planning, organization, and divided attention. The ECog has excellent test-retest reliability ($r = .82$) as well as strong convergent and discriminative validity when compared to other measures. For efficiency, the language and visuospatial ability subscales of the ECog were excluded in the current study. Specifically, the language section was considered unduly burdensome for older adults within the context of the larger assessment battery and its redundancy with screening questions (MATS) related to perceived word-finding difficulties. The visuospatial ability section was excluded as we did not perform any corroborative objective testing of visuospatial ability within our neuropsychological assessment. Thus, participants were only administered memory, planning, organization, and divided attention subscale items. Low scores on the ECog indicate worse functioning relative to same-aged peers, whereas high scores indicate better functioning relative to same-aged peers. The ECog is a commonly used measure in SCD studies and was considered a valuable inclusion in our analyses given our greater goal of identifying viable screening measures or items.

Memory and Aging Telephone Screen (MATS; Rabin et al., 2007). In addition to being used as a gross cognitive screening measure to determine eligibility alongside the MMSE-2, MATS responses were used to determine whether participants endorsed self-perceived changes in word-finding ability. Although word-finding challenges are typical of normative cognitive aging, declines in this area are commonly reported causes for distress among older adults. As such, it was deemed relevant to include the endorsement of word-finding declines in the regression analyses.

UCLA Loneliness Scale (Russell, Peplau, & Ferguson, 1978). In light of recent work demonstrating the unique accelerating effect of loneliness on cognitive decline (Donovan et al., 2017), it was considered important to include this variable in our regression analyses. Factor analysis has shown UCLA Loneliness Scale outcomes to be invariant with age and to be highly internally consistent (Ausín, Muñoz, Martín, Pérez-Santos, & Castellanos, 2019).

Neuropsychological assessment. The neuropsychological test battery was designed to closely parallel the Uniform Data Set used in the large-scale Alzheimer's Disease Neuroimaging

Initiative (ADNI) study (Weintraub et al., 2018). Lower than expected performance on neuropsychological measures was used to classify individuals as healthy controls or as demonstrating subtle CD.

Boston Naming Test, second edition (BNT; Kaplan, Goodglass, & Weintraub, 2000). The BNT is a measure of confrontation naming that is sensitive to disruptions in language. The BNT (or an abbreviated version) is commonly included in Alzheimer's research batteries (e.g., CERAD), as it has been shown to be sensitive to overall cognitive dysfunction (Mast & Gerstenecker, 2010).

California Verbal Learning Test, Second Edition (CVLT-2; Delis, Kramer, Kaplan, & Ober, 2000). The CVLT-2 measures verbal learning, retention, recall, and recognition. It further provides insight into executive functions, such as self-monitoring, inhibition (proneness to interference), and effort. Individuals with AD and other forms of objective cognitive impairment demonstrate clear and well-documented patterns of performance on the CVLT-2, making it an excellent diagnostic tool for objective cognitive decline (Gifford et al., 2015; Lezak, Howieson, Bigler, & Tranel, 2012).

Controlled Oral Word Association Test (COWAT; Ivnik et al., 1996). The COWAT is a test of verbal fluency, which includes aspects of executive functioning, word retrieval and processing speed (Lezak et al., 2012). As such, COWAT performance is sensitive to memory and prefrontal/executive deficits. Verbal fluency is not only sensitive to MCI, but the specific pattern of poor performance has been shown effective for differentiating specific pathologies (Price et al., 2012; Weakley, Schmitter-Edgecombe, & Anderson, 2013).

Golden Stroop Test (Stroop; Ivnik et al., 1996). The Stroop test provides insight into various cognitive functions, including processing speed, simple attention, word generation, and executive inhibition. Individuals with objective cognitive dysfunction, such as those with MCI and AD, have been found to perform more poorly than healthy controls on the inhibition task in particular (Bélanger, Belleville, & Gauthier, 2010).

Test of Practical Judgment (TOP-J; Rabin et al., 2007). The TOP-J is a measure designed to assess individuals' safety awareness and behaviours, problem-solving, and ability to navigate common daily activities. Owing to its' prefrontal/executive-loaded nature, the TOP-J has been shown to differentiate those with MCI, AD, and other objective cognitive impairment from cognitively intact individuals (Rabin et al., 2009). What is more, in the case that individuals are found to suffer from objective cognitive impairment, the TOP-J may provide insight into their relative safety in the community.

Trailmaking Test (TMT; Ivnik, Malec, Smith, Tangalos, & Petersen, 1996). Trailmaking Test A provides insight into simple attention, whereas Trailmaking Test B provides insight into selective attention, inhibition, and executive switching. Trailmaking Test B has been used to identify late-stage Alzheimer's disease and other prefrontal lobe dysfunction (Rapp & Reischies, 2005).

Wechsler Adult Intelligence Scale, fourth edition: Digit Span subtest (DS; Wechsler & Psychological Corporation, 2008). Digit span is a commonly used test in both clinical and research settings. Digit span-forward is a test of simple attention while digit span backward measures working memory. There is evidence that digit span is sensitive to MCI and may be sensitive to cognitive impairment among those with subjective memory complaints (Kurt, Yener, & Oguz, 2011). Analysis of reliable digit span may also be used as a measure of effort.

Wechsler Advanced Clinical Solution for the WAIS-IV and WMS-IV: Test of Premorbid Function (TOPF; Wechsler, 2008). The TOPF is commonly used in clinical and research settings to estimate premorbid cognitive ability based on demographic factors and performance on tasks insensitive to cognitive dysfunction (Wechsler, 2008). In the absence of comprehensive intelligence testing, The TOPF provides an estimate of individuals' premorbid intelligence. Where questions are raised regarding potential cognitive declines, TOPF performance may represent individuals' prior peak intellectual ability. This is determined using word reading ability, corrected for educational attainment and socioeconomic status.

Wechsler Memory Scale, fourth edition: Logical Memory subtest (LM; Wechsler & Psychological Corporation, 2008). In contrast to the CVLT-2, which assesses memory for non-contextual verbal information, the LM measures the influence of organization, meaning, and context on learning, retention, and recall.

Wechsler Memory Scale, fourth edition: Visual reproduction subtest (VR; Wechsler & Psychological Corporation, 2008). VM assesses individuals' learning and memory for non-verbal information. This test also provides opportunity for qualitative observation of fine motor functioning and frank visual disturbance.

Genetic sample collection. To obtain participants' APOE ε4 status, the Oragene OG-500 DNA saliva collection kit, mailable tube format, was used to obtain saliva samples from each participant. Oragene PrepIT L2P was used as a reagent for DNA extraction.

Outcomes

Binary logistic regression models for SCD endorsement and subtle CD resulting models are reported along with *p*-values, odds ratios per point increase, and 95% confidence intervals for odds ratio estimations per identified predictor.

Procedures

The study procedures were approved by the University of Victoria Human Research Ethics

Board and all activities were conducted in accordance with the Declaration of Helsinki. Following telephone screening and consent procedures, participants were administered paper-and-pencil questionnaires and asked to complete the measures independently. Upon completion, participants participated in a formal neuropsychological assessment administered by the Principal Investigator (JIA). Participants returned on a subsequent day to provide saliva samples and participate in an interview related to their perception of cognitive change with age (the results of which are reported elsewhere). Given the ethical concerns surrounding genetic status disclosure, as well as the uncertain nature of the meaning of SCD (Leuzy & Gauthier, 2012; Schicktanz et al., 2014; Tuokko & Smart, 2018), participants were not provided with the results of their neuropsychological assessment or genotype.

Analyses

Based on neuropsychological test performance, participants were coded as a healthy control or as demonstrating subtle CD. APOE ε4 genotype was determined via qPCR. The rs7412 and rs429358 single-nucleotide polymorphisms were isolated in order to discriminate between APOE ε2, ε3, and ε4 alleles. Participants carrying at least one APOE ε4 allele were considered to be APOE ε4-positive. All statistical analyses save for power analyses were performed using SPSS statistical software, Version 27.

Chi-squared analyses and independent samples *t*-tests were conducted to determine the equivalence of group demographic characteristics. As a preliminary step to our regression analyses, we performed bivariate two-way correlation analyses between all variables (criterion and predictor) to determine the extent of multicollinearity between variables. Following this, we conducted separate stepwise binary logistic regression analyses for each criterion variable (i.e., SCD endorsement, subtle CD). The order of entry for predictor variables into the model was determined according to the magnitude of effect. Removal of predictors was determined according to conditional parameter estimates of the likelihood ratio (i.e., Forward entry: Conditional). Those predictors with the greatest impact (based on the statistical significance of the effect) were entered first, followed by the next greatest contributor and so on in order until no further predictors were found to exert a significant influence on the criterion of interest.

Intended predictors were: 1) APOE ε4 genotype; 2) age; 3) sex; 4) education; 5) having a first-degree family member who is/was diagnosed with dementia; 6) having a current and/or historical diagnosis of psychological disorder (e.g., depression, anxiety); 7) self-reported decline in word-finding ability (MATS); 8) ECog memory subscale total t-score; 9) ECog organization subscale total t-score; 10) ECog planning subscale total t-score; 11) ECog divided attention subscale total t-score; 12) CCI total; 13) GDS total; 14) UCLA Loneliness Scale total; 15) AMAS-E worry/oversensitivity t-score; 16) AMAS-E physiological anxiety t-score; 17) AMAS-E fear of aging t-score; 18) AMAS-E lie scale t-score; 19) AMAS-E general (total) anxiety t-score. Additionally, 20) subtle CD was included as a predictor for SCD endorsement and *vice versa* to more directly test the relationship between subjective and potential objective cognitive decline. TOPF scores were found to be statistically invariant across groups. Further, TOPF outcomes are known to be significant influenced by education and socioeconomic status. Given its homogeneity, and partial determination by other established SCD contributors (e.g., education), the TOPF was excluded from the analyses in favour of other demographic factors. Limits were set to $p = .05$ for entry and $p=.10$ for removal from each model. Classification cut-off was set to 0.5.

Follow-up power analyses were conducted using G*Power version 3.1.9.7 software. Odds ratios (OR) were derived from the literature where possible. Where odds ratios were not available, an odds ratio of 1.5 was used instead. This was considered a conservative estimate based on the objective cognitive decline literature and an assumption of 10% change per unit. Analyses were calculated for power at different levels in order to provide a lower and upper range (0.40 and 0.70, respectively). Analyses were performed with an assumption of no covariates (i.e., predictor effects were considered in isolation). Given that no previous research on predictors/contributors to subtle CD were available, power analyses were conducted for SCD predictors separately.

Results

Sample Characteristics

Demographic data and self-report outcomes are provided in Table 3.1. The majority of our sample was comprised by retired professors, researchers, and university staff. Overall, the majority of our sample fell into the youngest-old/middle-old age group (M=73.92 years, SD=6.25 years), though a wide age range was represented (minimum=65 years, maximum=92 years). Our sample was relatively highly educated (M=15.85 years, SD=2.81 years) though, similarly, there was a wide range of educational achievement (minimum=8 years, maximum=20 years (PhD)). There was no significant difference between groups with regard to estimated premorbid intellectual functioning (TOPF); however, there was a trending (non-significant) difference between those with subtle CD and healthy controls (p=.051) such that those with subtle CD may have had slightly higher estimated premorbid intellectual ability. Paralleling age and education, the range in premorbid functioning estimates was large (minimum full-scale IQ (FSIQ) estimate=89, maximum FSIQ=127).

Subtle CD was demonstrated by 38.5% of the total sample (n=25/65). Participants demonstrating subtle CD were significantly younger than healthy controls (t=2.01, p=.049, Hedges' g=0.35) but did not significantly differ across any other demographic variable (e.g., APOE ε4 genotype, SCD endorsement, sex, years education, psychiatric diagnosis, first-degree family members with dementia). SCD was endorsed by 33.9% (n=22/65). Healthy controls endorsing SCD were less likely to have high cholesterol (χ^2=5.59, p=.018) versus healthy controls without concerns, however this did not translate to a significant overall difference between the healthy control and subtle CD groups. Groups were otherwise comparable across demographic variables.

Participants endorsed low depressive symptomology on the GDS (i.e., n=58 normal, n=7 mild) and this was invariant with group. All participants reported sub-clinical worry/oversensitivity and physiological anxiety on the AMAS-E; however, fear of aging ranged from subclinical to clinically significant (n=5/65, 7.7%). Lie scale scores remained within the expected range as did general (total) anxiety.

APOE ε4 Genotype Exclusion

As a well-established risk factor for neurodegeneration (Ali et al., 2018; Edmonds et al., 2015; Jessen, Wolfsgruber, et al., 2014) and a central variable of interest in this study, APOE ε4 genotype data was collected for all eligible participants. Unfortunately, the number of eligible participants recruited for this study was much lower than initially expected. As a result, the representation of APOE ε4-positive individuals in our sample was too low to perform meaningful group-level statistical comparisons (total n=11/65, 16.9%). APOE ε4-positive representation was diluted further still when divided across subtle CD and SCD status groups. In light of the low n of positive cases per group and consequently low power of APOE genotype as a predictor, this variable was excluded from the regression model calculations.

Correlation Analyses

The full correlation matrix is presented in full in Table 3.2. Correlation analyses indicated that our primary criterion variables, SCD endorsement and subtle CD, were not significantly related (r=0.04, p=.776), suggesting that they represent distinct constructs. Both criterion variables did, however, correlate with several predictor variables.

SCD endorsement was significantly associated with several measures of self-reported cognitive functioning, including word-finding difficulties (MATS: r=.317, p=.010), memory function relative to same-aged peers (ECog memory: r=-0.33, p=.007), and total cognitive decline (CCI: r=0.04, p=.776). It also correlated positively with anxiety related to physical functioning (AMAS-E physiological anxiety: r=0.26, p=.042), fear of aging and age-related changes (AMAS-E fear of aging: r=0.48, p<.001), and overall anxiety (AMAS-E general: r=0.29, p=.021), These correlations were consistent with the literature and aligned with expectations as SCD would, by definition, relate to perceived cognitive change and concern. More surprisingly, SCD endorsement was also associated with potential underreporting of anxiety (AMAS-E LIE: r=-0.27, p=.035) and lower endorsement of depressive symptoms (GDS: r=0.26, p=.034). It did not relate to any demographic factors.

In contrast, subtle CD related more closely to demographic factors than cognitive or psychosocial variables. With regard to self-perceived cognitive functioning, subtle CD only related to lower planning ability relative to same-aged peers (ECog planning: r=-0.32, p=.009). Demographically, subtle CD was inversely correlated with age (r=-0.25, p=.049) and having a first-degree family member with dementia (r=-0.35, p=.036). It did not significantly relate to any of our anxiety or depression measures.

The relationships between predictor variables were generally as expected. Subtests within a given measure correlated highly with each other, as did items within a similar domain (e.g, anxiety, depression, and positive psychiatric history). Overall, correlations between variables tended to fall below 0.7, the threshold beyond which multicollinearity would be expected to distort the regression model (Dormann et al., 2012).

Regression Analyses

Due to the exclusion of APOE ε4 genotype for low APOE ε4-positive representation, the final regression analyses for SCD endorsement and subtle CD were calculated using 20 potential predictors rather than the initially intended 21. See Tables 3.3 and 3.4 for a more detailed presentation of the final regression models for SCD endorsement and subtle CD, respectively.

SCD endorsement model.

First iteration. Performance of a binary logistic regression initially identified a seven-step model. Unique contributors to SCD endorsement in order of significance were identified as follow: 1) AMAS-E fear of aging *t*-score (*p*=.003, OR=1.35, CI 95%=1.11, 1.64); 2) having a first-degree relative with dementia (*p*=.029; OR=-0.07); 3) AMAS-E lie scale *t*-score (*p*=.032, OR=-0.89, CI 95%=0.80, 0.99); 4) self-endorsed word-finding decrements (*p*=.035; OR=14.96); 5) age (*p*=.037; OR=1.21; CI 95%=1.01, 1.45); 6) CCI total (*p*=.038; OR=1.16; CI 95%=1.01, 1.33); and 7) male sex (*p*=.063; OR=20.99). It should be noted that having a relative with dementia decreased the probability of SCD endorsement, whereas fear of aging, word-finding decrements, perceived cognitive change, and male sex each increased the probability of SCD endorsement. Further, those with SCD were more likely to over-report anxiety symptoms/concerns (AMAS-E lie scale) relative to their same-aged peers. This pattern of responding is frequently referred to as a "cry for help" profile and connotes a significant degree of emotional distress. The identified model improved the classification accuracy of the baseline model (i.e., including the intercept alone) from 66.2% to 87.7% overall. Correct identification of SCD specifically was increased from 0% to 81.80%. Further, the model explained a large proportion of unique variance contributing to SCD endorsement (Nagelkerke R^2=0.74); however, the inclusion of (male) sex as a predictor violated our predetermined significance threshold of α=.05.

Second iteration. The removal of participant sex as a predictor significantly (p=.011) changed the regression model. Recalculation of the regression excluding participant sex provided a six-step model: 1) AMAS-E fear of aging t-score (p=.003, OR=1.27, CI 95%=1.09, 1.47); 2) self-endorsed word-finding decrements (p=.023; OR=13.58); 3) having a first-degree relative with dementia (p=.024; OR=-0.10); 4) CCI total (p=.047; OR=1.12; CI 95%=1.00, 1.24); 5) AMAS-E lie scale t-score (p=.060, OR=-0.90, CI 95%=0.81, 1.01); and 6) age (p=.061; OR=1.16; CI 95%=0.99, 1.35). This model correctly classified 86.2% of individuals overall, 77.3% of those endorsing SCD. This model continued to explain a large proportion of unique variance contributing to SCD endorsement (Nagelkerke R^2=0.69); however, the removal of participant sex undermined the influence of AMAS-E lie scale t-score and participant age on SCD endorsement, leading their contribution to become non-significant. Follow-up t-tests did not support a significant effect of participant sex on age (t(63)=-.24, p=.808) or AMAS-E lie scale t-score (t(63)=.91, p=.367). Likewise, no significant correlation was found between age and AMAS-E lie scale t-score for male participants (Pearson's r=.084, p=.387). Unique among the identified predictors, having a relative with dementia continued to confer a significant protective effect.

Third iteration. The removal of AMAS-E lie scale t-score and participant age each significantly changed the regression model (p=.029, p=.042, respectively). Recalculation of the regression following the removal of these variables provided a four-step model: 1) AMAS-E fear of aging t-score (p=.003, OR=1.21, CI 95%=1.06, 1.37); 2) self-endorsed word-finding decrements (p=.030; OR=9.28); 3) CCI total (p=.042; OR=1.10; CI 95%=1.00, 1.20); and 4) having a first-degree relative with dementia (p=.053; OR=-0.20). The identified model correctly identified

81.5% of individuals overall and 72.7% of those endorsing SCD specifically. It explained a much-reduced proportion of the variance contributing to SCD endorsement relative to previous iterations (Nagelkerke R^2=0.56); however, the removal of the nonsignificant predictors from the previous model weakened the effect of having a first-degree relative with dementia. Follow-up t-test demonstrated no significant effect of participant sex on incidence of familial dementia (t(63)=1.06, p=.294).

Final iteration. The removal of having a first-degree relative with dementia as a predictor significantly changed the model (p=.034). Recalculation of the regression following the removal of first-degree relatives with dementia provided a final three-step model with significant predictors: 1) AMAS-E fear of aging t-score (p=.006, OR=1.16, CI 95%=1.04, 1.29); 2) self-endorsed word-finding decrements (p=.028; OR=8.44); and 3) CCI total (p=.035; OR=1.09; CI 95%=1.01, 1.18). The identified model correctly identified 76.9% of individuals overall; 86% of those with no concerns and 59.1% of those endorsing SCD. and the final model explained a moderate amount of the variance contributing to SCD endorsement (Nagelkerke R^2=0.50). All identified predictors conferred an increased risk of endorsing SCD. Variables excluded from the regression models included subtle CD, years of education, psychiatric diagnosis, generalized anxiety (AMAS-E worry/oversensitivity), anxiety regarding physical functioning and condition (AMAS-E physiological anxiety), depressive symptomology (GDS), loneliness (UCLA Loneliness Scale), and all ECog indices (memory, planning, organization, divided attention). None of the excluded variables were found to explain significant unique variance in SCD endorsement for any iteration of the model.

Subtle CD model. Only one iteration of the subtle CD model was calculated as the contributions of all identified predictors were significant. Regression analyses identified an optimized three-step solution. Significant predictors of subtle CD were identified as follow: 1) ECog planning mean score (p=.004; OR=-0.18; 95% CI=0.05, 0.58); 2) GDS total (p=.007; OR=-0.72; 95% CI=0.56, 0.91); and 3) AMAS-E physiological anxiety t-score (p=.015; OR=1.15; 95% CI=1.03, 1.28). This model improved the overall classification accuracy of the baseline model (i.e., including the intercept alone) from 66% to 78.5% of individuals with subtle CD. Correct identification of those with subtle CD increased from 0% to 56% in the final model. It should be noted that subtle CD was better identified by step 2 of the model (64%); however, a greater number of healthy controls were identified by the final step (92.5% as compared to 85% in step 2. The final model explained a relatively small amount of the unique variance (Nagelkerke R^2=0.34). Inverse to our expectations, higher depressive symptomology was associated with a decreased likelihood of demonstrating subtle CD. On the other hand, low self-reported planning ability (relative to peers) and high physiological anxiety conferred a greater risk of demonstrating subtle CD on objective tests. Notably, SCD was not identified as a significant predictor of subtle CD. Other variables excluded from the regression model included years of education, participant age, participant sex, having a first-degree relative with dementia, psychiatric diagnosis, self-reported word-finding difficulties (MATS), cognitive change (CCI), anxiety (AMAS-E worry/oversensitivity, fear of aging, physiological anxiety, total anxiety), response style (AMAS-E lie scale), loneliness (UCLA Loneliness Scale), and all ECog indices (memory, planning, organization, divided attention). None of the excluded variables were found to explain significant unique variance in SCD endorsement for any iteration of the model.

Power Analyses

In light of our low n and the unexpected exclusion of various theoretically-supported predictors from our SCD and subtle CD models, we determined that power analyses were warranted to clarify the sample size necessary to detect a significant effect for a given predictor. Our findings are summarized in Table 3.5.

With regard to our demographic variables, our sample of $n=65$ was confirmed to be underpowered for our regression analyses. For the sake of power analysis and lacking previously reports ORs, the majority of our dichotomous demographic predictors were estimated to increase the odds of SCD endorsement/subtle CD by 1.50 times when present. Based on these estimated values, a sample size of $n=191$ to $n=255$ would have been necessary in order to detect an effect with relatively low power (0.40). At a higher level of power (0.70), estimated necessary sample sizes exceeded $n=400$.

As may be expected, more data was available regarding the relationship between self-reported cognitive functioning and SCD. Further, measures like the ECog demonstrated a larger impact on SCD endorsement than our conservative estimates. Our sample size of $n=65$ exceeded the estimated sample necessary to detect an effect with weak power (0.40). It also met or exceeded the estimates for detecting effects of ECog memory, ECog planning, and ECog organization at a power of 0.70. However, our sample remained too small to detect changes at 0.70 for MATS word-finding ($n=127$), ECog divided attention ($n=77$), and CCI total ($n=127$).

Finally, with regard to psychosocial/mental health factors, our sample was within the acceptable range to detect effects of anxiety and loneliness at a power of 0.40, but was insufficient to detect significant effects of GDS or having a previous/current psychiatric diagnosis at the same level of power. Similar outcomes were found at our higher power estimate (0.70).

Discussion

The aims of this study were several. First, we sought to 1) determine whether and which combination of psychosocial factors, demographic variables, APOE ε4 genotype, and low cognitive performance corresponded to SCD endorsement. In turn, our second aim was to 2) determine whether and which combination of psychosocial factors, demographic variables, APOE ε4 genotype, and SCD aligned with low cognitive performance.

APOE ε4 Genotype

Before ensuing a comprehensive review of our identified regression models, the under-representation of APOE ε4-positive genotype warrants some consideration. It has been shown that carriers of the APOE ε4 allele may be at increased risk of experiencing SCD and neurodegeneration (e.g., Ali et al., 2018; Edmonds et al., 2015; Herrmann et al., 2019). Despite our attempt to include APOE ε4 genotype as a key predictor, however, there were too few positive cases (*n*=11/65, 16.9%) to perform meaningful statistical analyses of any possible genetic contribution to SCD or subtle CD in our sample. Although the absolute number of APOE ε4-positive cases was low, it bears mentioning that the proportion of APOE ε4-positive individuals in our sample was roughly equivalent to what would be expected for our population of healthy older adults with primarily Northern European origin. For instance, McKay and colleagues estimated that approximately 13% of European adults between the ages of 66 and 90 years carry the APOE ε4 allele (McKay et al., 2011) while Kern and coworkers estimated a prevalence of approximately 15.6% in their comparable community sample (Kern et al., 2015). For context, the prevalence of APOE ε4 genotype among AD samples may surpass 60% (Ward et al., 2012). Given the proportional representation of APOE ε4 genotype in our sample, the low frequency of APOE ε4 genotype in our sample is likely due to a small *n* overall.

SCD Contributors

Early iterations. Although our final model was relatively robust, some of the earlier SCD models may merit attention. Initial analyses identified male sex as the single greatest factor contributing to SCD endorsement (i.e., increasing the odds of SCD endorsement over 20x versus being female) despite participant sex failing to reach statistical significance as a predictor. This is notable given our relatively small sample of male participants (n=14). Subsequent removal of this variable from our model had a cascading effect on the contributions of age, distress/"cry for help" responding, and the influence of having a first-degree relative with dementia. Follow-up t-tests failed to substantiate any direct effect of participant sex on the contributions of participant age, distress, or familial dementia; however, the trending effect of participant sex (p=.063) despite the low n of males (14/65) suggests that this variable may simply have had inadequate power to reach statistical significance.

Culling these non-significant predictors from our model led to a final solution where all contributors exerted a significant degree of unique influence over SCD endorsement; however this final model performed more poorly than our initial iteration with respect to correctly identifying endorsers. Our first model (with non-significant predictors included) correctly classified 81.8% of SCD endorsers, whereas our final model correctly classified 59.1% of SCD endorsers. Although our final model may present the most robust predictors of SCD endorsement, it is likely that a number of the removed non-significant predictors may also have added explanatory value. Unfortunately, the forward entry method we employed for our regression analyses prioritizes the uniqueness of a given predictor's contribution. The culled predictors may still be important considerations for screening purposes.

Final model. Several iterations of our SCD model were calculated due to the inclusion of non-significant contributors. Our final model identified fear of aging (AMAS-E), self-endorsed word-finding declines (MATS), and overall cognitive decline (CCI) as the variables with the most significant unique impacts on SCD endorsement. Our final solution aligns with the literature and suggests that SCD in our community sample may more reliably reflect anxiety amidst relatively normative age-related cognitive changes than measurable pathological decline.

The principle role of anxiety – specifically anxiety related to age-related changes – in SCD endorsement was consistent with expectations given the previous implication of anxious distress and trait neuroticism in at least some cases of SCD/cognitive complaint endorsement (Haavisto, 2018; Merema, Speelman, Foster, & Kaczmarek, 2013; Pearman & Storandt, 2005; Snitz et al., 2015). For instance, a recent review by Hill and coworkers (Hill et al., 2016) found anxiety to be "consistently associated" with subjective cognitive impairments (i.e, SCD). This is not to say, however, that anxiety necessarily causes SCD endorsement in a unidirectional fashion. Tobiansky and colleagues (Tobiansky, Livingston, & Mann, 1995) present a case for a reciprocal relationship between anxiety symptoms and SCD. In their longitudinal study, it was found that older adults with SCD were not only more likely to endorse anxiety symptoms at baseline, but that they were also more likely to endorse increasing anxious symptomology over time. Similarly, other work has found anxiety to predispose individuals toward SCD but also to increase in turn when individuals perceived their cognitive abilities to decline (Hill et al., 2019; Verhaeghen, Geraerts, & Marcoen, 2000). Importantly, Rabin, Smart, and Amariglio (2017) caution against discounting this interaction as purely "worry feeding worry". In at least some cases, it remains distinctly possible that SCD and coincident anxiety represent emergent manifestations of inchoate neuropathological processes.

Regardless of the specific cause of perceived decline, a key factor in the relationship between anxiety and SCD may be attunement or vigilance to one's cognitive functioning. It is possible that those who endorse SCD may be particularly attuned to perturbations in their cognitive functioning and, perhaps, most likely to translate these into global fears regarding aging and age-related changes to life and ability. If so, it may be expected those who demonstrate more self-focused attention report SCD more often. Further, it may be that highly-educated individuals (e.g., those whose professional/personal identities may relate most closely to their cognitive functioning) would be exceedingly sensitive to reporting SCD. Indeed, both of these hypotheses have been supported in the literature (self-focused attention: Chin, Oh, Seo, & Na, 2014; education effects: Tuokko & Smart, 2018; van Oijen, de Jong, Hofman, Koudstaal, & Breteler, 2007). Given that our sample was relatively homogeneous, it is unsurprising that educational achievement did not explain unique variance in our model of SCD endorsement. Though it is difficult to speculate, it is considered probable that education may have been a more prominent predictor of SCD in a more educationally diverse sample.

Interestingly, general worry and overall anxiety were not identified as significant predictors. The identification of fear of aging as key predictor was distinct. To our knowledge, this is not a finding that has been reported previously. Among our sample of highly educated, community-based retired professionals, SCD appeared to be a manifestation of attunement to and discomfort around normative age-related cognitive change, rather than an expression of dementia concerns *per se*. This was reinforced during our intake and qualitative follow-ups (discussed in detail in a subsequent study) where our sample demonstrated an idiosyncratic interpretation of cognitive concern that was disparate from the majority of SCD literature. When those with SCD were asked to elaborate on their concerns, almost all stated that they were concerned about their general cognitive decline over time and the potential for developing dementia in the far future. Importantly, these participants believed strongly that they were currently functioning well – in many cases, even better than their same-aged peers – and that their concerns were normative given their stage of life. Taking the above into account, and in line with the unique found effect of fear of aging, our findings appear to support Hill et al.'s conclusion that the most salient driver of the anxiety-SCD relationship may be underlying fears related to loss of (independent) function (Hill et al., 2016).

Excluded variables. Although the prevailing evidence appears to support our model's inclusion of fear of aging as a predictor, the exclusion of depression (GDS) from our models would appear more anomalous. Depression is arguably the most consistently identified corollary of SCD. For instance, a review by Brigola and coworkers demonstrated that the severity of subjective memory complaints was associated with depression and affective factors more than objective functioning across numerous studies (Brigola et al., 2015). Relevant to the current study, Zlatar and colleagues' found that GDS score was positively associated with SCD endorsement (Zlatar et al., 2018); however, this may have been partly inflate by the endorsement of specific GDS items related to perceived cognitive change. Other work has identified depression and SCD as independent and multiplicative risk factors for objective cognitive decline (Liew, 2019; Rabin, Smart, & Amariglio, 2017). Despite the well-established influence of depression on SCD, range restriction in our sample's GDS ratings may have undermined any possible effects. Specifically, only n=7 participants rated their depressive symptoms above the "mild depression" threshold, and none in the "moderate depression" or "severe depression" range. This outcome was invariant in our sample regardless of whether the GDS total score was calculated with cognitive change-related items excluded. It is probable that, given a larger and more diverse sample, depression may have been identified as a more salient and significant predictor.

Other unexpected model exclusions were the ECog domain-specific subscale totals. Upon review, it was evident that each ECog subscale suffered from relatively severe restrictions in the range of represented scores. With very few exceptions, participants in our sample indicated that their cognitive functioning was comparable or superior to same-aged others across all cognitive domains. It is quite possible that the functional and concrete nature of ECog items may not have been optimal for identifying the sub-clinical subjective changes experienced by those endorsing SCD. Those with SCD would not be expected to experience significant disruption in daily activities and, thus, may not have resonated with the specific declines listed in the measure. Yet another contributor to the discordance between ECog ratings and SCD endorsement may have been the misfit of the ECog with our operational definition of SCD. We predicated our classification of SCD on the self-reporting of cognitive concern, a key feature of Jessen et al.'s criteria for high-risk SCD *Plus* (Jessen, Amariglio, et al., 2014). Specifically, we asked individuals whether they perceived any declines from their own cognitive baseline that cause concern. The ECog response options, on the other hand, are framed in terms of how well individuals feel they perform specific cognitive tasks relative to same-aged others. This is an important distinction as our sample consisted primarily of former academics and professionals who – often very explicitly – reported a degree of pride in their intellect and cognitive functioning relative to their peers. When cognitive concerns were raised, participants frequently clarified that they still believed they continued to function "better" than others but that they were frustrated by perceived declines in their abilities relative to what they believed they were capable of when they were younger. Despite the ECog's relatively frequent inclusion in SCD research (Rabin et al., 2015), the crucial element of fit with SCD criteria and definition may influence a number of outcomes. Reliance on the ECog as a measure of self-perceived cognitive functioning may be misguided when SCD is defined as a purely intrapersonal construct and/or when a sample is likely to be highly educated. This discrepancy may also explain why the CCI, which measures self-perceived change in ability, related to SCD endorsement when the ECog subscales did not.

Perhaps the most poignant exclusion from our final model was subtle CD, our proxy for burgeoning objective decline in cognitive functioning. While it is true that stepwise regression models occasionally overlook important contributing variables due to their lack of uniqueness, subtle CD was not indicated even when other identified predictors were factored out of the model. It is possible that subtle CD represented a rate of change that was too early in its progression, too subtle to be observed, or too common to be considered troubling by participants. Indeed, the relatively high base rate of older adults achieving scores >1 SD below the age-normative mean (Binder et al., 2009) suggests that subtle CD may not be a sensitive enough indicator of objective cognitive decline or neuropathological risk. This may be further supported by Edmonds and coworkers' own findings that subtle CD was most predictive of objective dysfunction when paired with amyloidosis and/or neurodegeneration (Edmonds et al., 2015).

Subtle CD Contributors

With regard to objective 2), self-reported decrements in planning ability, *lower* depressive symptomology, and higher anxiety regarding physiological changes were the strongest predictors of subtle CD. The inclusion of planning ability may be especially interesting in light of the historical trend for cognitive risk literature to include or focus primarily on episodic memory functioning as a primary predictor (Hamel et al., 2015; Ying Lim et al., 2013). Departing from this, our findings suggest that the self-reported ease and efficacy of complex frontal-executive abilities may be a more sensitive index of subtle neurological disruption at the earliest stages. Indeed, this conclusion aligns with the sentiments of the SCD-I Working Group, who specifically advocate for the use of "cognitive" rather than "memory" when discussing SCD because memory may not be the first domain to decline across all neurodegenerative processes, despite its salience in amnestic MCI and Alzheimer's disease (Jessen, 2014; Smart & Krawitz, 2015).

Perhaps more surprising were the seemingly protective effects of age and depressive symptomology. Both advanced age and depression are regularly identified as strong risk factors for pathological cognitive decline and dementia conversion (Heser et al., 2013; Sachs-Ericsson et al., 2014); however, our sample appeared to differ in this regard. Since there is no evidence among the SCD, aging, or dementia literature to suggest that relative youth should be riskier in any regard, it is most likely that the observed effect of age may reflect the characteristics of our self-selected sample more than incipient cognitive impairment *per se*. Specifically, it is entirely possible that participants of more advanced age chose to participate in the study due to their confidence in their cognitive abilities, whereas those younger opted to join out of concern or curiosity regarding their functioning. While speculative, this interpretation would align well with the oldest-old participants' reported reasons for participating during intake versus the youngest-old. On the other hand, the protective effect of depressive symptomology may be more emblematic of a response bias among older adults experiencing more objective – if sub-clinical – changes in cognitive and daily functioning. It is well-established that older adults display a positivity bias, whereby individuals tend to disengage from fear- or anxiety-provoking stimuli in order to regulate potential emotional distress (e.g., Lee & Knight, 2009; Xing & Isaacowitz, 2006). Combined with the face valid nature of GDS items, those particularly suspicious of objective cognitive changes may have been less likely to acknowledge any frank emotional distress on our depression measure. In light of evidence that GDS scores historically correlate positively with SCD endorsement (Zlatar et al., 2018), this contrary relationship with subtle CD supports the conclusion that SCD and subtle CD are separable constructs.

Yet another somewhat surprising significant risk indicator was self-reported anxiety related to physiological functioning. At first glance, the inclusion of physiological anxiety may seem entirely unrelated to the cognitive interests of this study; however, for many older adults, physiological functioning and cognitive functioning may load onto a unitary construct, that of functional independence. Where fear of aging in general was a predictor of SCD endorsement, those experiencing lower cognitive performance currently (i.e., subtle CD) likely experience and express more salient concerns related to their autonomy. Since the AMAS-E does not include a subscale devoted to cognitive functioning in particular, challenges to autonomy and independence are addressed most directly by items devoted to issues with mobility, accessibility, and physical health.

Caveats, Limitations, and Future Recommendations

Our models identified a number of variables that may herald SCD and, potentially, subtle CD. While valuable, these models do warrant several qualifications. The low representation of APOE ε4 genotype and its subsequent exclusion from our analyses has been addressed above. Another caveat that may merit further discussion, however, is the specific interpretation of cognitive concern and SCD across our sample. Risk-conferring SCD is characterized as self-reported declines in cognitive functioning paired with concern that these changes are pathological or, at least, beyond what one would expect given an individual's age (Jessen et al., 2020). Despite our efforts to abide by SCD classification methods used previously by credible large-scale studies (i.e., single item querying concern regarding perceived cognitive declines (Rabin, Smart, & Amariglio, 2017), our participants uniformly reported that their concerns related to the abstract possibility of developing dementia in the far future rather than any belief that their current experience reflected a pathological process. Few of our SCD-endorsing participants believed that their current functioning was indicative of pathology and none had sought formal medical advice or assistance to mitigate these changes as a result. Beyond the various challenges of comparing data from clinical SCD samples and community-based SCD samples reported exhaustively elsewhere (Abdelnour et al., 2017; Rodríguez-Gómez, Abdelnour, Jessen, Valero, & Boada, 2015; Snitz et al., 2018), this nuanced interpretation of "concern" in our study raises questions regarding the invariance, efficacy, and overall validity of single-item SCD classification methods.

Related, our self-selected sample may have represented a sub-population of the older adult community that was less likely to experience and/or report SCD, despite our specific recruitment for persons with SCD. As noted above, our sample almost wholly consisted of individuals whose professional identities centred around their cognitive abilities and who – according to participant self-disclosures –were relatively confident in the superiority of their functioning relative to same-aged peers. In fact, some participants reported that their associates with more pronounced cognitive concerns were the least interested in participating in our study due to fears that their concerns would be reinforced.

Together, this suggests that the current study may have preferentially appealed to older adults with a distinct aging experience and, potentially, fewer underlying cognitive risk factors. Consequently, our findings may not be entirely generalizable to older adults as a whole or even those who are most anxious about perceived cognitive decrements. Nevertheless, the described models may be particularly useful for predicting subtle and early risk among those older adults most likely to present for general medical check-up; that is, those who do not yet have marked concerns about their functioning but who are exceedingly vigilant to changes in their cognition and/or physiological functioning.

Another, more statistical, consideration is the large number of predictor variables included in both of the regression models fit for this study. We included 19 variables per model (excluding APOE ε4 genotype). This number is admittedly large, especially considering the commonly cited "one-in-ten" convention to prevent overfitting of models, whereby one predictor is recommended for every ten events and the number of events are determined by the smallest of the outcome categories (Harrell, Lee, & Mark, 1996). However, this rule-of-thumb has been called into question for being too conservative. For instance, Austin and Steyerberg (2015) have demonstrated that as few as two subjects per variable may provide an adequately unbiased estimation of regression coefficients, standard errors, and confidence intervals. Vittinghoff and McCulloch (2007) reinforce this finding, demonstrating that sample size exerts little to no influence on the accuracy of confidence interval estimates. Additionally, we felt it acceptable to contravene the conventional statistical wisdom for the purposes of the current investigation. Specifically, the goals for this study were exploratory rather than confirmatory in nature. Given the novelty of our work, we deemed it suitable to include a larger number of variables at this initial stage of research so that future iterations may benefit from a targeted list of predictors likely to exert a significant influence.

However, although we were successful in identifying several variables that may be most likely to influence SCD endorsement/subtle CD, our low n did undermine our statistical power – that is, our ability to detect other effects that may also have been important. Specifically, our power analyses demonstrated that we would not have been able to detect any effects of depressive symptomology or other demographic variables regardless of their influence. These are important exclusions as the current literature supports depression, age, and education as key contributors to SCD endorsement and objective decline alike. The inclusion of such a large number of predictors may also have impacted the sensitivity of our analyses. Model entry was determined based on the significant *unique* influence of a given predictor on our criterion variables (i.e., SCD endorsement, subtle CD). Although our potential predictors were theoretically supported and derived, the effect of individual variables may have been diluted among so many others. Essentially, our variables may have "competed" with one another. As a result, it is possible that our analyses may have overlooked other important variables that contributed explanatory value but that were not unique among the other predictors in the field.

Finally, subtle CD served as a proxy for potential sub-clinical cognitive performance decrements in our sample of healthy older adults. Although the NIA-AA (Sperling et al., 2011) and Edmonds and colleagues (2015) determined that subtle CD may provide an early indication of cognitive and functional decline, it remains unclear whether the Edmonds criteria is diagnostically sound. For instance, Binder et al. (2009) discuss the typicality of achieving low scores across comprehensive test batteries. In contrast to Edmonds et al. (2015), Binder et al. (2009) demonstrate that achieving as many as six scores >1 standard deviation below the age-normative mean is relatively common among older adults (i.e., >5% base rate). While individuals with higher educational achievement are expected to demonstrated somewhat fewer low scores (Binder et al., 2009), it remains unclear exactly what a clinically meaningful frequency threshold for dementia risk might actually be. With this in mind, it is difficult to discern whether our general adherence to Edmonds et al.'s (2015) subtle CD criteria was too sensitive to normal test score variance or too insensitive to potential underlying neuropathology. Further, without longitudinal follow-up, it is impossible to know whether our assumption of cognitive risk is substantiated in the longer term.

Future iterations of this work would benefit from a larger and more ethnically, socioeconomically, educationally, and sexually diverse sample. It would be challenging to recruit individuals based on genetic biomarker diversity but it is expected that a more representative sample in other respects might reflect more variation in genetic risk as well. Further, direct comparison of clinical and community-based samples with SCD would help to clarify which predictors may be specific to the construct of interest vs. avoidance/help-seeking inclination. In light of the potential shortcomings of single-item SCD determination and evidence suggesting that SCD classification may differ depending on assessment method (Vogel, Salem, Andersen, & Waldemar, 2016), it may be useful for future large-scale studies to include multiple potential determinants of SCD. Identifying predictors of SCD according to various metrics and tracking objective cognitive outcomes longitudinally may provide the best evidence for how to discern risk-conferring SCD from normative age-related cognitive concerns. As a precursor, a reliability analysis of various SCD classification methods may be warranted. Due to the unclear diagnostic value of (potential) subtle CD, it would also be valuable to compare those with differing degrees (e.g., two low scores vs. three vs. four) and patterns of (potential) subtle CD to clarify potential risk thresholds. Unfortunately, the current study's sample did not demonstrate significant enough variation in the number of low scores or the specific cognitive domains/measures with low scores to perform any meaningful analysis. Finally, the current study excluded the language and visuospatial ability sections of the ECog measure as several language items were redundant with data already collected and few corresponding objective visuospatial tests were administered. However, in light of previous findings that self-reported visuospatial processing deficits might be particularly predictive of eventual objective cognitive impairment (Amariglio, Townsend, Grodstein, Sperling, & Rentz, 2011), this decision may have been imprudent. The inclusion of the entire ECog (or a parallel self-reported cognitive function measure) in future work may be recommended to allow more comprehensive analysis of the particular domains of self-perceived change linked with objective decline as well as the calculation of a total ECog score.

Conclusions

As a whole, our models indicate that SCD endorsement is not necessarily associated with objective cognitive decrements in their potential earliest developmental phase. Instead, SCD may reflect perceived declines in word-finding and general cognitive functioning, as well as overarching anxiety regarding the aging process. There is also evidence to suggest that, when older men are open to reporting about their cognitive performance, they may be more likely than older woman to endorse SCD. Given previous findings, it is likely that depression and educational achievement may each play a more prominent role in SCD endorsement; however, isolating the contribution of these variables was not possible given our small and relatively homogeneous sample (e.g., range restriction). On the other hand, subtle CD, a presumed and potential precursor to objective cognitive impairments, may be detected somewhat accurately by querying older adults about observed changes in planning ability, depressive symptomology, and concerns regarding current/future health and physiological functioning. These findings support the contention of the SCD-I working group that non-memory cognitive domains, such as executive functioning, may present a more sensitive index of incipient neuropathological decline. Taken together, our findings demonstrate that SCD and subtle (objective) cognitive decline are separable constructs that may contribute uniquely to overall function and diagnostic status in later life.

Funding

This work was supported by the Alzheimer Society of Canada (Dr. & Mrs. Albert Spatz Award, 18-29) and the Lou-Poy family via the University of Victoria Institute on Aging and Lifelong Health (Alice Lou-Poy Graduate Scholarship).

References

Abdelnour, C., Rodríguez-Gómez, O., Alegret, M., Valero, S., Moreno-Grau, S., Sanabria, Á., …

Boada, M. (2017). Impact of recruitment methods in subjective cognitive decline. *Journal
of Alzheimer's Disease : JAD*, *57*(2), 625–632. https://doi.org/10.3233/JAD-160915

Ali, J. I., Smart, C. M., & Gawryluk, J. R. (2018). Subjective cognitive decline and APOE E4: A
systematic review. *Journal of Alzheimer's Disease*, *65*(1), 303–320.

Allan, C. L., & Ebmeier, K. P. (2011). The influence of ApoE4 on clinical progression of
dementia: A meta-analysis. *International Journal of Geriatric Psychiatry*, *26*(5), 520–526.
https://doi.org/10.1002/gps.2559

Allaz, A.-F., & Cedraschi, C. (2015). *Emotional aspects of chronic pain*. In G. Pickering & S.
Gibson (Eds.), *Pain, Emotion and Cognition: A Complex Nexus* (pp. 21–34). New York,
NY: Springer.

Amariglio, R. E., Becker, J. A., Carmasin, J., Wadsworth, L. P., Lorius, N., Sullivan, C., …
Rentz, D. M. (2012). Subjective cognitive complaints and amyloid burden in cognitively
normal older individuals. *Neuropsychologia*, *50*(12), 2880–2886.
https://doi.org/10.1016/j.neuropsychologia.2012.08.011

Amariglio, R. E., Townsend, M. K., Grodstein, F., Sperling, R. A., & Rentz, D. M. (2011).
Specific subjective memory complaints in older persons may indicate poor cognitive
function. *Journal of the American Geriatrics Society*, *59*(9), 1612–1617.
https://doi.org/10.1111/j.1532-5415.2011.03543.x

Ausín, B., Muñoz, M., Martín, T., Pérez-Santos, E., & Castellanos, M. Á. (2019). Confirmatory
factor analysis of the Revised UCLA Loneliness Scale (UCLA LS-R) in individuals over
65. *Aging and Mental Health*, *23*(3), 345–351.

https://doi.org/10.1080/13607863.2017.1423036

Austin, P. C., & Steyerberg, E. W. (2015). The number of subjects per variable required in linear

regression analyses. *Journal of Clinical Epidemiology, 68*(6), 627–636.

https://doi.org/10.1016/j.jclinepi.2014.12.014

Balash, Y., Mordechovich, M., Shabtai, H., Giladi, N., Gurevich, T., & Korczyn, A. D. (2013).

Subjective memory complaints in elders: Depression, anxiety, or cognitive decline?. *Acta

Neurologica Scandinavica, 127*, 344–350.

Bélanger, S., Belleville, S., & Gauthier, S. (2010). Inhibition impairments in Alzheimer's

disease, mild cognitive impairment and healthy aging: Effect of congruency proportion in a

Stroop task. *Neuropsychologia, 48*(2), 581–590.

https://doi.org/10.1016/j.neuropsychologia.2009.10.021

Binder, L. M., Iverson, G. L., & Brooks, B. L. (2009). To err is human: "Abnormal"

neuropsychological scores and variability are common in healthy adults. *Archives of

Clinical Neuropsychology, 24*(1), 31–46. https://doi.org/10.1093/arclin/acn001

Brigola, A. G., Manzini, C. S. S., Oliveira, G. B. S., Ottaviani, A. C., Sako, M. P., & Vale, F. A.

C. (2015). Subjective memory complaints associated with depression and cognitive

impairment in the elderly: A systematic review. *Dementia & Neuropsychologia, 9*(1), 51–

57. https://doi.org/10.1590/s1980-57642015dn91000009

Buckley, R. F., Villemagne, V. L., Masters, C. L., Ellis, K. A., Rowe, C. C., Johnson, K., …

Amariglio, R. (2016). A conceptualization of the Utility of subjective cognitive decline in

clinical trials of preclinical Alzheimer's disease. *Journal of Molecular Neuroscience, 60*(3),

354–361. https://doi.org/10.1007/s12031-016-0810-z

Chen, K.-L., Sun, Y.-M., Zhou, Y., Zhao, Q.-H., Ding, D., & Guo, Q.-H. (2016). Associations between APOE polymorphisms and seven diseases with cognitive impairment including Alzheimer's disease, frontotemporal dementia, and dementia with Lewy bodies in southeast China. *Psychiatric Genetics, 26*(3), 124–131. https://doi.org/10.1097/YPG.0000000000000126

Cherbuin, N., Sargent-Cox, K., Easteal, S., Sachdev, P., & Anstey, K. J. (2015). Hippocampal atrophy is associated with subjective memory decline: The PATH Through Life Study. *American Journal of Geriatric Psychiatry, 23*(5), 546–556. https://doi.org/10.1016/j.jagp.2014.07.009

Chin, J., Oh, K. J., Seo, S. W., & Na, D. L. (2014). Are depressive symptomatology and self-focused attention associated with subjective memory impairment in older adults?. *International Psychogeriatrics, 26*(4), 573–580. https://doi.org/10.1017/S104161021300241X

Comijs, H. C., Deeg, D. J. H., Dik, M. G., Twisk, J. W. R., & Jonker, C. (2002). Memory complaints; the association with psycho-affective and health problems and the role of personality characteristics. A 6-year follow-up study. *Journal of Affective Disorders, 72*(2), 157–165. https://doi.org/10.1016/S0165-0327(01)00453-0

Cooper, C., Bebbington, P., Lindesay, J., Meltzer, H., McManus, S., Jenkins, R., & Livingston, G. (2011). The meaning of reporting forgetfulness: A cross-sectional study of adults in the English 2007 Adult Psychiatric Morbidity Survey. *Age and Ageing, 40*(6), 711–717. https://doi.org/10.1093/ageing/afr121

Delis, D. C., Kramer, J. H., Kaplan, E., & Ober, B. A. (2000). *California Verbal Learning Test, Second Edition*. San Antonio, TX: Pearson.

Derouesné, C., Lacomblez, L., Thibault, S., & LePoncin, M. (1999). Memory complaints in young and elderly subjects. *International Journal of Geriatric Psychiatry, 14*(4), 291–301.

https://doi.org/10.1002/(SICI)1099-1166(199904)14:4<291::AID-GPS902>3.0.CO;2-7

Diefenbach, G. J., Bragdon, L. B., & Blank, K. (2014). Geriatric Anxiety Inventory: Factor

structure and associations with cognitive status. *The American Journal of Geriatric*

Psychiatry, 22(12), 1418–1426.

Donovan, N. J., Wu, Q., Rentz, D. M., Sperling, R. A., Marshall, G. A., & Glymour, M. M.

(2017). Loneliness, depression and cognitive function in older U.S. adults. *International*

Journal of Geriatric Psychiatry, 32(5), 564–573. https://doi.org/10.1002/gps.4495

Dormann, C. F., Elith, J., Bacher, S., Buchmann, C., Carl, G., Carré, G., … Lautenbach, S.

(2012). Collinearity: A review of methods to deal with it and a simulation study evaluating

their performance. *Ecography, 36*(1), 27–46.

Dux, M. C., Woodard, J. L., Calamari, J. E., Messina, M., Arora, S., Chik, H., & Pontarelli, N.

(2008). The moderating role of negative affect on objective verbal memory performance

and subjective memory complaints in healthy older adults. *Journal of the International*

Neuropsychological Society: JINS, 14(2), 327–336.

https://doi.org/10.1017/S1355617708080363

Edmonds, E. C., Delano-Wood, L., Galasko, D. R., Salmon, D. P., & Bondi, M. W. (2015).

Subtle cognitive decline and biomarker staging in preclinical Alzheimer's disease. *Journal*

of Alzheimer's Disease, 47(1), 231–242. https://doi.org/10.3233/JAD-150128

Farias, S. T., Mungas, D., Reed, B. R., Cahn-Weiner, D., Jagust, W., Baynes, K., & DeCarli, C.

(2008). The Measurement of Everyday Cognition (ECog): Scale development and

psychometric properties. *Neuropsychology, 22*(4), 531–544. https://doi.org/10.1037/0894-

4105.22.4.531

Farrer, L. A., Cupples, A. L., Kukull, W. a, Mayeux, R., Myers, R. H., Pericak-vance, M. a, …

van Duijn, C. M. (1997). Effects of age , sex , and ethnicity on the association between

apolipoprotein E genotype and Alzheimer disease. *JAMA: The Journal of the American

Medical Association, 278*, 1349–1356. https://doi.org/10.1001/jama.1997.03550160069041

Fonseca, J. A. S., Ducksbury, R., Rodda, J., Whitfield, T., Nagaraj, C., Suresh, K., … Walker, Z.

(2015). Factors that predict cognitive decline in patients with subjective cognitive

impairment. *International Psychogeriatrics/IPA, 27*(10), 1671–1677.

https://doi.org/10.1017/S1041610215000356

Fortea, J., Sala-Llonch, R., Bartrés-Faz, D., Lladó, A., Solé-Padullés, C., Bosch, B., … Rami, L.

(2011). Cognitively preserved subjects with transitional cerebrospinal fluid β-amyloid 1-42

values have thicker cortex in Alzheimer's disease vulnerable areas. *Biological Psychiatry,

70*(2), 183–190. https://doi.org/10.1016/j.biopsych.2011.02.017

Gibson, S. J. (2015). The pain, emotion and cognition nexus in older persons and in dementia. In

G. Pickering & S. Gibson (Eds.), *Pain, Emotion and Cognition: A Complex Nexus* (pp. 231–

247). New York, NY: Springer.

Gifford, K. A., Bell, S. P., Liu, D., Neal, J. E., Turchan, M., Shah, A. S., & Jefferson, A. L.

(2019). Frailty is related to subjective cognitive decline in older women with dementia.

Journal of the American Geriatrics Society, 67(9), 1803–1811.

Gifford, K. A., Liu, D., Damon, S. M., Chapman, W. G., Romano, R. R., Samuels, L. R., …

Jefferson, A. L. (2015). Subjective memory complaint only relates to verbal episodic

memory performance in mild cognitive impairment. *Journal of Alzheimer's Disease, 44*(1),

309–318. https://doi.org/10.3233/JAD-140636

Goesling, J., Clauw, D. J., & Hassett, A. L. (2013). Pain and depression: An integrative review

of neurobiological and psychological factors. *Current Psychiatry Reports, 15*(12), 421.
https://doi.org/10.1007/s11920-013-0421-0

Haavisto, W. (2018). Do individual differences explain discrepancies between subjective
memory and objective memory? *book Abstracts International Section A: Humanities and
Social Sciences, 79*(1-A).

Hamel, R., Köhler, S., Sistermans, N., Koene, T., Pijnenburg, Y., Van Der Flier, W., …
Ramakers, I. (2015). The trajectory of cognitive decline in the pre-dementia phase in
memory clinic visitors: Findings from the 4C-MCI study. *Psychological Medicine, 45*(7),
1509–1519. https://doi.org/10.1017/S0033291714002645

Harrell, F. E., Lee, K. L., & Mark, D. B. (1996). Multivariable prognostic models: Issues in
developing models, evaluating assumptions and adequacy, and measuring and reducing
errors. *Statistics in Medicine, 15,* 361–387. https://doi.org/10.1002/(SICI)1097-
0258(19960229)15:4<361::AID-SIM168>3.0.CO;2-4

Herrmann, F. R., Rodriguez, C., Haller, S., Garibotto, V., Montandon, M. L., & Giannakopoulos,
P. (2019). Gray matter densities in limbic areas and APOE4 independently predict cognitive
decline in normal brain aging. *Frontiers in Aging Neuroscience, 11,* 157.
https://doi.org/10.3389/fnagi.2019.00157

Heser, K., Tebarth, F., Wiese, B., Eisele, M., Bickel, H., Köhler, M., … Age CoDe Study Group.
(2013). Age of major depression onset, depressive symptoms, and risk for subsequent
dementia: Results of the German study on Ageing, Cognition, and Dementia in Primary
Care Patients (AgeCoDe). *Psychological Medicine, 43*(8), 1597–1610.
https://doi.org/10.1017/S0033291712002449

Hill, N. L., Mogle, J., Bell, T. R., Bhargava, S., Wion, R. K., & Bhang, I. (2019). Predicting current and future anxiety symptoms in cognitively intact older adults with memory

complaints. *International Journal of Geriatric Psychiatry, 34*(12), 1874–1882.

https://doi.org/10.1002/gps.5204

Hill, N. L., Mogle, J., Wion, R., Munoz, E., DePasquale, N., Yevchak, A. M., & Parisi, J. M.

(2016). Subjective cognitive impairment and affective symptoms: A systematic review.

Gerontologist, 56(6), e109–e127. https://doi.org/10.1093/geront/gnw091

Imtiaz, B., Tolppanen, A. M., Kivipelto, M., & Soininen, H. (2014). Future directions in

Alzheimer's disease from risk factors to prevention. *Biochemical Pharmacology, 88*(4),

661–670. https://doi.org/10.1016/j.bcp.2014.01.003

Ivnik, R. J., Malec, J. F., Smith, G. E., Tangalos, E. G., & Petersen, R. C. (1996).

Neuropsychological tests' norms above age 55: COWAT, BNT, MAE token, WRAT-R

reading, AMNART, STROOP, TMT, and JLO. *The Clinical Neuropsychologist, 10*(3),

262–278. https://doi.org/10.1080/13854049608406689

Jack, C. R., Bennett, D. A., Blennow, K., Carrillo, M. C., Dunn, B., Haeberlein, S. B., …

Silverberg, N. (2018). NIA-AA Research Framework: Toward a biological definition of

Alzheimer's disease. *Alzheimer's and Dementia, 14*(4), 535–562.

https://doi.org/10.1016/j.jalz.2018.02.018

Jenkins, A., Tree, J. J., Thornton, I. M., & Tales, A. (2019). Subjective cognitive impairment in

55-65-year-old adults is associated with negative affective symptoms, neuroticism, and poor

quality of life. *Journal of Alzheimer's Disease, 67*(4), 1367–1378.

https://doi.org/10.3233/JAD-180810

Jessen, F. (2014). Subjective and objective cognitive decline at the pre-dementia stage of

Alzheimer's disease. *European Archives of Psychiatry and Clinical Neuroscience, 264*(1),

3–7. https://doi.org/10.1007/s00406-014-0539-z

Jessen, F., Amariglio, R. E., Buckley, R. F., van der Flier, W. M., Han, Y., Molinuevo, J. L., … Wagner, M. (2020). The characterisation of subjective cognitive decline. *The Lancet Neurology*, *19*(3), 271–278. https://doi.org/10.1016/S1474-4422(19)30368-0

Jessen, F., Amariglio, R. E., Van Boxtel, M., Breteler, M., Ceccaldi, M., Chételat, G., … Wagner, M. (2014). A conceptual framework for research on subjective cognitive decline in preclinical Alzheimer's disease. *Alzheimer's and Dementia*, *10*(6), 844–852. https://doi.org/10.1016/j.jalz.2014.01.001

Jessen, F., Wiese, B., Cvetanovska, G., Fuchs, A., Kaduszkiewicz, H., Kölsch, H., … Bickel, H. (2007). Patterns of subjective memory impairment in the elderly: Association with memory performance. *Psychological Medicine*, *37*(12), 1753–1762. https://doi.org/10.1017/S0033291707001122

Jessen, F., Wolfsgruber, S., Wiese, B., Bickel, H., Mösch, E., Kaduszkiewicz, H., … Wagner, M. (2014). AD dementia risk in late MCI, in early MCI, and in subjective memory impairment. *Alzheimer's and Dementia*, *10*(1), 76–83. https://doi.org/10.1016/j.jalz.2012.09.017

Jiang, S., Tang, L., Zhao, N., Yang, W., Qiu, Y., & Chen, H. Z. (2016). A systems view of the differences between APOE ε4 carriers and non-carriers in Alzheimer's disease. *Frontiers in Aging Neuroscience*, *8*, 171. https://doi.org/10.3389/fnagi.2016.00171

Jonker, C., Geerlings, M. I., & Schmand, B. (2000). Are memory complaints predictive for dementia? A review of clinical and population-based studies. *International Journal of Geriatric Psychiatry*, *15*(11), 983–991. https://doi.org/10.1002/1099-1166(200011)15:11<983::aid-gps238>3.0.co;2-5

Kaplan, E., Goodglass, H., & Weintraub, S. (2000). *Boston Naming Test, Second Edition*. San

Antonio, TX: Pearson.

Kern, S., Mehlig, K., Kern, J., Zetterberg, H., Thelle, D., Skoog, I., … Börjesson-Hanson, A. (2015). The distribution of apolipoprotein e genotype over the adult lifespan and in relation to country of birth. *American Journal of Epidemiology, 181*(3), 214–217. https://doi.org/10.1093/aje/kwu442

Kim, S., Kim, M. J., Kim, S., Kang, H. S., Lim, S. W., Myung, W., … Kim, D. K. (2015). Gender differences in risk factors for transition from mild cognitive impairment to Alzheimer's disease: A CREDOS study. *Comprehensive Psychiatry, 62,* 114–122. https://doi.org/10.1016/j.comppsych.2015.07.002

Krell-Roesch, J., Woodruff, B. K., Acosta, J. I., Locke, D. E., Hentz, J. G., Stonnington, C. M., … Geda, Y. E. (2015). APOE ε4 genotype and the risk for subjective cognitive impairment in elderly persons. *The Journal of Neuropsychiatry and Clinical Neurosciences, 27*(4), 322–325. https://doi.org/10.1176/appi.neuropsych.14100268

Kurt, P., Yener, G., & Oguz, M. (2011). Impaired digit span can predict further cognitive decline in older people with subjective memory complaint: A preliminary result. *Aging & Mental Health, 15*(3), 364–369. https://doi.org/10.1080/13607863.2010.536133

Lee, L. O., & Knight, B. G. (2009). Attentional bias for threat in older adults: Moderation of the positivity bias by trait anxiety and stimulus modality. *Psychology and Aging, 24*(3), 741–747. https://doi.org/10.1037/a0016409

Leuzy, A., & Gauthier, S. (2012). Ethical issues in Alzheimer's disease: An overview. *Expert Review of Neurotherapeutics, 12*(5), 557–567. https://doi.org/10.1586/ern.12.38

Lezak, M. D., Howieson, D. B., Bigler, E. D., & Tranel, D. (2012). *Neuropsychological assessment, fifth edition.* New York, NY: Oxford University Press.

Liew, T. M. (2019). Depression, subjective cognitive decline, and the risk of neurocognitive

disorders. *Alzheimer's Research and Therapy, 11*, 70. https://doi.org/10.1186/s13195-019-

0527-7

Lista, S., Molinuevo, J. L., Cavedo, E., Rami, L., Amouyel, P., Teipel, S. J., … Hampel, H.

(2015). Evolving evidence for the value of neuroimaging methods and biological markers in

subjects categorized with subjective cognitive decline. *Journal of Alzheimer's Disease,

48*(S1), S171–S191. https://doi.org/10.3233/JAD-150202

Liu, Y., Tan, L., Wang, H.-F., Liu, Y., Hao, X.-K., Tan, C.-C., … Alzheimer's Disease

Neuroimaging Initiative. (2016). Multiple effect of APOE genotype on clinical and

neuroimaging biomarkers across Alzheimer's disease spectrum. *Molecular Neurobiology,

53*(7), 4539–4547. https://doi.org/10.1007/s12035-015-9388-7

Lowe, P. A., & Raad, J. M. (2006). Psychometric analyses of the AMAS-E scores in a sample of

older adults. *Individual Differences Research, 4*(4), 272–290.

Lowe, P. A., & Reynolds, C. R. (2006). Examination of the psychometric properties of the Adult

Manifest Anxiety Scale-Elderly Version Scores. *Educational and Psychological

Measurement, 66*(1), 93–115. https://doi.org/10.1177/0013164405278563

Mast, B. T., & Gerstenecker, A. (2010). Screening instruments and brief batteries for dementia.

In P. A. Lichtenberg (Ed.), *Handbook of Assessment in Clinical Gerontology, Second

Edition* (pp. 503–530). Cambridge, MS: Academic Press.

Mata, I. F., Leverenz, J. B., Weintraub, D., Trojanowski, J. Q., Hurtig, H. I., Van Deerlin, V. M.,

… Zabetian, C. P. (2014). APOE, MAPT, and SNCA genes and cognitive performance in

Parkinson disease. *JAMA Neurology, 71*(11), 1405–1412.

https://doi.org/10.1001/jamaneurol.2014.1455

McKay, G. J., Silvestri, G., Chakravarthy, U., Dasari, S., Fritsche, L. G., Weber, B. H., …

Patterson, C. C. (2011). Variations in apolipoprotein e frequency with age in a pooled

analysis of a large group of older people. *American Journal of Epidemiology, 173*(12),

1357–1364. https://doi.org/10.1093/aje/kwr015

Merema, M. R., Speelman, C. P., Foster, J. K., & Kaczmarek, E. A. (2013). Neuroticism (not

depressive symptoms) predicts memory complaints in some community-dwelling older

adults. *American Journal of Geriatric Psychiatry, 21*(8), 729–736.

https://doi.org/10.1016/j.jagp.2013.01.059

Müller-Gerards, D., Weimar, C., Abramowski, J., Tebrügge, S., Jokisch, M., Dragano, N., …

Winkler, A. (2019). Subjective cognitive decline, APOE ε4, and incident mild cognitive

impairment in men and women. *Alzheimer's and Dementia: Diagnosis, Assessment and

Disease Monitoring, 11,* 221–230. https://doi.org/10.1016/j.dadm.2019.01.007

Pearman, A., & Storandt, M. (2005). Self-discipline and self-consciousness predict subjective

memory in older adults. *Journals of Gerontology: Series B Psychological Sciences and

Social Sciences, 60*(3), P153–P157. https://doi.org/10.1093/geronb/60.3.P153

Pérès, K., Helmer, C., Amieva, H., Matharan, F., Carcaillon, L., Jacqmin-Gadda, H., …

Dartigues, J. F. (2011). Gender differences in the prodromal signs of dementia: Memory

complaint and IADL-restriction. A prospective population-based cohort. *Journal of

Alzheimer's Disease, 27*(1), 39–47. https://doi.org/10.3233/JAD-2011-110428

Perrotin, A., Mormino, E. C., Madison, C. M., Hayenga, A. O., & Jagust, W. J. (2012).

Subjective Cognition and Amyloid Deposition Imaging: A Pittsburgh Compound B Positron

Emission Tomography Study in Normal Elderly Individuals. *Archives of Neurology, 69*(2),

223–229. https://doi.org/10.1001/archneurol.2011.666

Pink, A., Stokin, G. B., Bartley, M. M., Roberts, R. O., Sochor, O., Machulda, M. M., … Geda, Y. E. (2015). Neuropsychiatric symptoms, APOE ε4, and the risk of incident dementia: A population-based study. *Neurology, 84*(9), 935–943. https://doi.org/10.1212/WNL.0000000000001307

Prestia, A., Caroli, A., Wade, S. K., van der Flier, W. M., Ossenkoppele, R., Van Berckel, B., … Frisoni, G. B. (2015). Prediction of AD dementia by biomarkers following the NIA-AA and IWG diagnostic criteria in MCI patients from three European memory clinics. *Neuropsychology Review, 11*(10), 1191–1201. https://doi.org/10.1016/j.jalz.2014.12.001

Price, S. E., Kinsella, G. J., Ong, B., Storey, E., Mullaly, E., Phillips, M., … Perre, D. (2012). Semantic verbal fluency strategies in amnestic mild cognitive impairment. *Neuropsychology, 26*(4), 490–497. https://doi.org/10.1037/a0028567

Rabin, L. A., Borgos, M. J., Saykin, A. J., Wishart, H. A., Crane, P. K., Nutter-Upham, K. E., & Flashman, L. A. (2007). Judgment in older adults: Development and psychometric evaluation of the Test of Practical Judgment (TOP-J). *Journal of Clinical and Experimental Neuropsychology, 29*(7), 752–767. https://doi.org/10.1080/13825580601025908

Rabin, L. A., Saykin, A. J., West, J. D., Borgos, M. J., Wishart, H. A., Nutter-Upham, K. E., … Santulli, R. B. (2009). Judgment in older adults with normal cognition, cognitive complaints, MCI, and mild AD: Relation to regional frontal gray matter. *Brain Imaging and Behavior, 3*(2), 212–219. https://doi.org/10.1007/s11682-009-9063-6

Rabin, L. A., Saykin, A. J., Wishart, H. A., Nutter-Upham, K. E., Flashman, L. A., Pare, N., & Santulli, R. B. (2007). The Memory and Aging Telephone Screen: Development and preliminary validation. *Alzheimer's and Dementia, 3*(2), 109–121. https://doi.org/10.1016/j.jalz.2007.02.002

Rabin, L. A., Smart, C. M., & Amariglio, R. E. (2017). Subjective cognitive decline in

preclinical Alzheimer's disease. *Annual Review of Clinical Psychology, 13*(1), 369–396.

https://doi.org/10.1146/annurev-clinpsy-032816-045136

Rabin, L. A., Smart, C. M., Crane, P. K., Amariglio, R. E., Berman, L. M., Boada, M., … Sikkes,

S. A. M. (2015). Subjective cognitive decline in older adults: An overview of self-report

measures used across 19 international research studies. *Journal of Alzheimer's Disease,*

48(S1), S63–S86. https://doi.org/10.3233/JAD-150154

Rapp, M. A., & Reischies, F. M. (2005). Attention and executive control predict Alzheimer

disease in late life: Results from the Berlin Aging Study (BASE). *American Journal of*

Geriatric Psychiatry, 13(2), 134–141. https://doi.org/10.1097/00019442-200502000-00007

Rattanabannakit, C., Risacher, S. L., Gao, S., Lane, K. A., Brown, S. A., McDonald, B. C., …

Farlow, M. R. (2016). The Cognitive Change Index as a measure of self and informant

perception of cognitive decline: Relation to neuropsychological tests. *Journal of*

Alzheimer's Disease, 51(4), 1145–1155. https://doi.org/10.3233/JAD-150729

Reisberg, B., Shulman, M. B., Torossian, C., Leng, L., & Zhu, W. (2010). Outcome over seven

years of healthy adults with and without subjective cognitive impairment. *Neuropsychology*

Review, 6(1), 11–24. https://doi.org/10.1016/j.jalz.2009.10.002

Reynolds, C. R., Richmond, B. O., Lowe, P. A. (2003). *Adult Manifest Anxiety Scale*. Torrance,

CA: Western Psychological Services.

Rodríguez-Gómez, O., Abdelnour, C., Jessen, F., Valero, S., & Boada, M. (2015). Influence of

sampling and recruitment methods in studies of subjective cognitive decline. *Journal of*

Alzheimer's Disease, 48(S1), S99–S107. https://doi.org/10.3233/JAD-150189

Russell, D., Peplau, L. A., & Ferguson, M. L. (1978). Developing a measure of loneliness.

Journal of Personality Assessment, 42(3), 290–294.

https://doi.org/10.1207/s15327752jpa4203_11

Sachs-Ericsson, N., Moxley, J. H., Corsentino, E., Rushing, N. C., Sheffler, J., Selby, E. A., … Steffens, D. C. (2014). Melancholia in later life: Late and early onset differences in presentation, course, and dementia risk. *International Journal of Geriatric Psychiatry, 29*(9), 943–951. https://doi.org/10.1002/gps.4083

Saykin, A. J., Wishart, H. A., Rabin, L. A., Santulli, R. B., Flashman, L. A., West, J. D., … Mamourian, A. C. (2006). Older adults with cognitive complaints show brain atrophy similar to that of amnestic MCI. *Neurology, 67*(5), 834–842. https://doi.org/10.1212/01.wnl.0000234032.77541.a2

Scerri, C. (2014). The curvy side of dementia: The impact of gender on prevalence and caregiving. *Journal of the Malta College of Pharmacy Practice, 20*, 37–39.

Schicktanz, S., Schweda, M., Ballenger, J. F., Fox, P. J., Halpern, J., Kramer, J. H., … Jagust, W. J. (2014). Before it is too late: Professional responsibilities in late-onset Alzheimer's research and pre-symptomatic prediction. *Frontiers in Human Neuroscience, 8*, 921. https://doi.org/10.3389/fnhum.2014.00921

Shaw, S., & Hoeber, L. (2003). "A strong man is direct and a direct woman is a bitch": Gendered discourses and their influence on employment roles in sports organizations. *Journal of Sport Management, 17*(4), 347–376.

Slavin, M. J., Brodaty, H., Kochan, N. A., Crawford, J. D., Trollor, J. N., Draper, B., & Sachdev, P. S. (2010). Prevalence and predictors of "subjective cognitive complaints" in the Sydney Memory and Ageing Study. *American Journal of Geriatric Psychiatry, 18*(8), 701–710. https://doi.org/10.1097/JGP.0b013e3181df49fb

Smart, C. M., Karr, J. E., Areshenkoff, C. N., Rabin, L. A., Hudon, C., Gates, N., … Wesselman,

   L. (2017). Non-Pharmacologic interventions for older adults with subjective cognitive

   decline: Systematic review, meta-analysis, and preliminary recommendations.

   Neuropsychology Review, 27(3), 245–257. https://doi.org/10.1007/s11065-017-9342-8

Smart, C. M., & Krawitz, A. (2015). The impact of subjective cognitive decline on Iowa

   Gambling Task performance. *Neuropsychology, 29*(6), 971–987.

   https://doi.org/10.1037/neu0000204

Snitz, B. E., Lopez, O. L., McDade, E., Becker, J. T., Cohen, A. D., Price, J. C., … Klunk, W. E.

   (2015). Amyloid-β imaging in older adults presenting to a memory clinic with subjective

   cognitive decline: A pilot study. *Journal of Alzheimer's Disease, 48*(S1), S151–S159.

   https://doi.org/10.3233/JAD-150113

Snitz, B. E., Wang, T., Cloonan, Y. K., Jacobsen, E., Chang, C. C. H., Hughes, T. F., … Ganguli,

   M. (2018). Risk of progression from subjective cognitive decline to mild cognitive

   impairment: The role of study setting. *Alzheimer's and Dementia, 14*(6), 734–742.

   https://doi.org/10.1016/j.jalz.2017.12.003

Sperling, R. A., Aisen, P. S., Beckett, L. A., Bennett, D. A., Craft, S., Fagan, A. M., … Phelps,

   C. H. (2011). Toward defining the preclinical stages of Alzheimer's disease:

   Recommendations from the National Institute on Aging-Alzheimer's Association

   workgroups on diagnostic guidelines for Alzheimer's disease. *Alzheimer's and Dementia,*

   7(3), 280–292. https://doi.org/10.1016/j.jalz.2011.03.003

Stern, Y. (2012). Cognitive reserve in ageing and Alzheimer's disease. *The Lancet Neurology,*

   11(11), 1006–1012.

Stewart, R., Russ, C., Richards, M., Brayne, C., Lovestone, S., & Mann, A. (2001). Depression,

APOE genotype and subjective memory impairment: A cross-sectional study in an African-Caribbean population. *Psychological Medicine, 31*(3), 431–440.

Stewart, R., Godin, O., Crivello, F., Maillard, P., Mazoyer, B., Tzourio, C., & Dufouil, C. (2011). Longitudinal neuroimaging correlates of subjective memory impairment: 4-year prospective community study. *British Journal of Psychiatry, 198*(3), 199–205. https://doi.org/10.1192/bjp.bp.110.078683

Tandetnik, C., Hergueta, T., Bonnet, P., Dubois, B., & Bungener, C. (2017). Influence of early maladaptive schemas, depression, and anxiety on the intensity of self-reported cognitive complaint in older adults with subjective cognitive decline. *International Psychogeriatrics, 29*(10), 1657–1667.

Tobiansky, R., Livingston, G., & Mann, A. (1995). The Gospel Oak Study stage IV: The clinical relevance of subjective memory impairment in older people. *Psychological Medicine, 25*(4), 779–786. https://doi.org/10.1017/S0033291700035029

Tomita, T., Sugawara, N., Kaneda, A., Okubo, N., Iwane, K., Takahashi, I., … Yasui-Furukori, N. (2014). Sex-specific effects of subjective memory complaints with respect to cognitive impairment or depressive symptoms. *Psychiatry and Clinical Neurosciences, 68*(3), 176–181. https://doi.org/10.1111/pcn.12102

Tuokko, H. A., & Smart, C. M. (2018). *Neuropsychology of cognitive decline: A developmental approach to assessment and intervention.* New York, NY: Guilford Press.

van Oijen, M., de Jong, F. J., Hofman, A., Koudstaal, P. J., & Breteler, M. M. B. (2007). Subjective memory complaints, education, and risk of Alzheimer's disease. *Alzheimer's and Dementia, 3*(2), 92–97. https://doi.org/10.1016/j.jalz.2007.01.011

Verhaeghen, P., Geraerts, N., & Marcoen, A. (2000). Memory complaints, coping, and well-being in old age: A systemic approach. *Gerontologist, 40*(5), 540–548.

https://doi.org/10.1093/geront/40.5.540

Vittinghoff, E., & McCulloch, C. E. (2007). Relaxing the rule of ten events per variable in

logistic and cox regression. *American Journal of Epidemiology, 165*(6), 710–718.

https://doi.org/10.1093/aje/kwk052

Vogel, A., Salem, L. C., Andersen, B. B., & Waldemar, G. (2016). Differences in quantitative

methods for measuring subjective cognitive decline - Results from a prospective memory

clinic study. *International Psychogeriatrics, 28*(9), 1513–1520.

https://doi.org/10.1017/S1041610216000272

Ward, A., Crean, S., Mercaldi, C. J., Collins, J. M., Boyd, D., Cook, M. N., & Arrighi, H. M.

(2012). Prevalence of apolipoprotein E4 genotype and homozygotes (APOE e4/4) among

patients diagnosed with Alzheimer's disease: A systematic review and meta-analysis.

Neuroepidemiology, 38(1), 1–17. https://doi.org/10.1159/000334607

Weakley, A., Schmitter-Edgecombe, M., & Anderson, J. (2013). Analysis of verbal fluency

ability in amnestic and non-amnestic mild cognitive impairment. *Archives of Clinical

Neuropsychology, 28*(7), 721–731. https://doi.org/10.1093/arclin/act058

Wechsler, D. (2008). *Wechsler Advanced Clinical Solutions for the WAIS-IV and WMS-IV*. San

Antonio, TX: Pearson.

Wechsler, D., & Psychological Corporation. (2008). *Wechsler Memory Scale, Fourth Edition*.

San Antonio, TX: The Psychological Corporation.

Weintraub, S., Besser, L., Dodge, H. H., Teylan, M., Ferris, S., Goldstein, F. C., … Morris, J. C.

(2018). Version 3 of the Alzheimer Disease Centers' neuropsychological test battery in the

Uniform Data Set (UDS). *Alzheimer Disease and Associated Disorders, 32*(1), 10–17.

https://doi.org/10.1097/WAD.0000000000000223

Xing, C., & Isaacowitz, D. M. (2006). Aiming at happiness: How motivation affects attention to and memory for emotional images. *Motivation and Emotion, 30*(3), 249–256. https://doi.org/10.1007/s11031-006-9032-y

Yesavage, J. A., Brink, T. L., Rose, T. L., Lum, O., Huang, V., Adey, M., & Leirer, V. O. (1982). Development and validation of a geriatric depression screening scale: A preliminary report. *Journal of Psychiatric Research, 17*(1), 1982–1983. https://doi.org/10.1016/0022-3956(82)90033-4

Ying Lim, Y., Ellis, K. A., Harrington, K., Kamer, A., Pietrzak, R. H., Bush, A. I., … Maruff, P. (2013). Cognitive consequences of high aβ amyloid in mild cognitive impairment and healthy older adults: Implications for early detection of Alzheimer's disease. *Neuropsychology, 27*(3), 322–332. https://doi.org/10.1037/a0032321

Zlatar, Z. Z., Muniz, M. C., Espinoza, S. G., Gratianne, R., Gollan, T. H., Galasko, D., & Salmon, D. P. (2018). Subjective cognitive decline, objective cognition, and depression in older Hispanics screened for memory impairment. *Journal of Alzheimer's Disease, 63*(3), 949–956. https://doi.org/10.3233/JAD-170865

Tables

Table 3.1. Participant demographics and psychosocial variables

	Healthy Control n=40			Subtle CD n=25			HC vs. Subtle
	No Concern n=27	SCD n=13	p-value	No Concern n=16	SCD n=9	p-value	p-value
General							
Female n (%)	21 (77.78)	11 (84.62)	.613	12 (75.00)	7 (77.78)	.876	.703
Age M (SD)	74.96 (6.41)	75.46 (7.63)	.830	70.19 (4.45)	75.22 (4.12)	**.010**	**.049**
Yrs Education M (SD)	16.15 (2.71)	16.31 (2.29)	.856	15.00 (3.16)	15.78 (3.23)	.564	.201
TOPF: Estimated general intelligence M (SD)	110.31 (10.57)	112.75 (8.82)	.491	105.56 (8.64)	107.11 (10.59)	.695	.051
Genetic Risk							
APOE ε4-positive n (%)	4 (14.82)	2 (15.38)	.962	2 (12.50)	3 (33.33)	.211	.601
Family dementia Hx n (%)	10 (37.04)	9 (69.23)	.056	5 (31.25)	2 (22.22)	.629	.118
Mental Health Hx							
Depression n (%)	7 (25.93)	5 (38.46)	.418	4 (25.00)	2 (22.22)	.876	.599
Anxiety n (%)	3 (11.11)	1 (7.69)	.736	1 (6.25)	2 (22.22)	.238	.800
PTSD n (%)	1 (3.70)	1 (7.69)	.588	0 (0.00)	0 (0.00)	-	-
Physical Health Hx							
Cancer n (%)	5 (18.52)	5 (38.46)	.172	4 (25.00)	3 (33.33)	.656	.789
Diabetes n (%)	4 (14.82)	1 (7.69)	.523	1 (6.25)	1 (11.11)	.667	.569
Heart problems n (%)	7 (25.93)	3 (23.08)	.845	2 (12.50)	0 (0.00)	.269	.086
High blood pressure n (%)	7 (25.93)	4 (30.77)	.748	2 (12.50)	1 (11.11)	.918	.139
High cholesterol n (%)	9 (33.33)	0 (0.00)	**.018**	2 (12.50)	1 (11.11)	.918	.288
Psychosocial Factors							
UCLA Loneliness Scale: Total loneliness M (SD)	11.07 (8.10)	14.08 (11.18)	.339	11.56 (10.21)	13.89 (12.25)	.615	.889
GDS: Total depression M (SD)	4.33 (4.19)	6.00 (4.20)	.246	2.50 (2.97)	5.56 (3.25)	**.025**	.205
AMAS-E: Worry/oversensitivity M (SD)	45.59 (7.28)	45.46 (8.44)	.973	43.50 (8.35)	48.22 (8.12)	.184	.859
AMAS-E: Physiological anxiety M (SD)	42.04 (6.12)	44.69 (9.18)	.354	43.25 (6.81)	49.11 (6.55)	**.047**	.168
AMAS-E: Fear of aging M (SD)	45.96 (7.34)	53.08 (8.42)	**.016**	44.50 (7.20)	56.56 (6.54)	***<001***	.721
AMAS-E: Lie scale M (SD)	49.41 (8.40)	45.69 (8.10)	.152	54.25 (9.71)	47.67 (6.80)	.086	.098
AMAS-E: General (total) anxiety M (SD)	43.96 (7.31)	46.77 (8.27)	.320	42.50 (9.12)	50.67 (6.23)	**.026**	.761
Self-reported Cognitive Change/Functioning							
MATS: Word-finding difficulties n (%)	14 (51.85)	11 (84.62)	**.045**	12 (75.00)	9 (36.00)	.102	.064
CCI: Total cognitive change M (SD)	31.48 (6.76)	39.85 (11.21)	***.006***	33.25 (7.73)	40.22 (10.56)	.070	.510
ECog: Memory M (SD)	3.59 (0.52)	3.26 (0.50)	.069	3.55 (0.54)	3.09 (0.61)	.061	.491
ECog: Planning M (SD)	4.13 (0.52)	4.05 (0.67)	.654	3.84 (0.56)	3.51 (0.47)	.154	**.009**
ECog: Organization M (SD)	3.75 (0.69)	3.96 (0.65)	.370	3.84 (0.89)	3.48 (0.82)	.328	.582
ECog: Divided attention M (SD)	3.67 (0.70)	3.31 (0.79)	.154	3.38 (0.84)	3.14 (0.45)	.369	.169

Bold-face: Significant at p<.05; ***Bold-face italic***: Significant at p<.01

Table 3.2. Bivariate two-way correlations (*Pearson's r*)

	Criterion		Predictor																	
	SCD	Subtle CD	Age	Sex	Education	TOPF	Family w/Dementia	Psych. Dx	MATS Word-finding	ECog Memory	ECog Planning	ECog Organization	ECog Divided Attn.	CCI	GDS	UCLA Loneliness	AMAS-E WOS	AMAS-E PHYS	AMAS-E FEAR	AMAS-E LIE	AMAS-E GENERAL
SCD	-																				
Subtle CD	.04	-																			
Age	.17	**-.25**	-																		
(Male) Sex	-.06	.05	.03	-																	
Education	.06	-.16	.02	.14	-																
TOPF	.09	-.25	.08	.03	**.52**	-															
Family w/Dementia	.06	**-.35**	-.18	-.20	.31	.13	-														
Psych. Dx	.13	-.01	.01	-1.2	.06	.04	-.14	-													
MATS Word-finding	**.32**	.23	-.17	-.08	.16	-.13	-.04	.01	-												
ECog Memory	**-.33**	-.09	**.25**	.07	-.09	-.22	-.07	-.16	-.09	-											
ECog Planning	-.16	**-.32**	.17	-.13	.08	-.07	.16	-.10	-.05	**.59**	-										
ECog Organization	-.01	-.07	.12	-.05	.13	-.05	.01	.09	.04	**.58**	**.65**	-									
ECog Divided Attn.	-.21	-.17	-.06	-.04	.02	-.21	-.03	-.14	.04	**.49**	**.62**	**.31**	-								
CCI	**.41**	.08	.06	.24	.01	.04	-.01	.08	.08	**-.41**	**-.38**	-.16	**-.31**	-							
GDS	**.26**	-.16	-.04	.03	.21	**.34**	.19	**.27**	-.07	**-.29**	-.21	-.09	**-.30**	**.40**	-						
UCLA Loneliness	.13	.02	-.10	.01	.11	-.01	.20	**.30**	.03	-.08	.02	.21	-.18	.17	**.42**	-					
AMAS-E WOS	.11	-.02	-.05	.01	.03	-.01	.05	**.27**	-.11	-.11	-.04	.11	.02	**.25**	**.48**	**.36**	-				
AMAS-E PHYS	**.26**	.18	.03	.11	.13	.21	.02	**.26**	.07	-.20	-.08	-.03	.06	**.46**	**.54**	**.26**	**.52**	-			
AMAS-E FEAR	**.50**	.05	.06	.17	.15	.02	.08	-.01	.22	**-.28**	-.12	-.06	-.04	**.36**	**.28**	.16	**.51**	**.42**	-		
AMAS-E LIE	**-.27**	.21	-.17	-.11	-.12	**-.31**	-.03	-.01	-.05	.08	-.09	-.14	.15	-.10	-.17	-.11	.03	-.09	.05	-	
AMAS-E GENERAL	**.29**	.04	-.04	.06	.13	.10	.04	.23	.06	-.23	-.10	.09	.05	**.38**	**.50**	**.31**	**.90**	**.72**	**.72**	.02	-

Bold-face: Significant at *p*<.05; ***Bold-face italic***: Significant at *p*<.01

190

Table 3.3 SCD endorsement regression model

Predictors/Outcomes	β	SE	Wald	df	p-value	Odds Ratio	95% CI for OR	Significance of change if removed
Step 0								
Constant	-0.67	0.26	6.54	1	.011	0.51	-	-
Overall classification accuracy=66.20%								
No Concern=100.00%								
SCD=0.00%								
Step 1								
AMAS-E fear of aging	0.16	0.05	12.03	1	.001	1.18	1.07, 1.29	<.001
Constant	-8.78	2.40	13.36	1	<.001	0.00	-	-
Nagelkerke R²=0.34								
Overall accuracy=70.80%								
No Concern=79.10%								
SCD=54.50%								
Step 2								
MATS word-finding decline	1.91	0.91	4.42	1	.036	6.74	1.14, 39.90	.015
AMAS-E fear of aging	0.17	0.05	10.89	1	.001	1.18	1.07, 1.31	<.001
Constant	-10.52	2.83	13.87	1	<.001	0.00	-	-
Nagelkerke R²=0.43								
Overall accuracy=73.80%								
No Concern=86.00%								
SCD=50.00%								
Step 3								
MATS word-finding decline	2.13	0.97	4.82	1	.028	8.44	1.26, 56.68	.010
CCI total cognitive decline	0.08	0.04	4.47	1	.035	1.09	1.01, 1.18	.022
AMAS-E fear of aging	0.15	0.05	7.66	1	.006	1.16	1.04, 1.29	.001
Constant	-12.768	3.26	15.35	1	<.001	0.00	-	-
Nagelkerke R²=0.50								
Overall accuracy=76.9%								
No Concern=86.00%								
SCD=59.10%								

Table 3.4 Subtle CD regression model

Predictors/Outcomes	β	SE	Wald	df	*p*-value	Odds Ratio	95% CI for OR	Significance of change if removed
Step 0								
Constant	-0.47	0.26	3.40	1	.065	0.63	-	-
Overall classification accuracy=61.50%								
Healthy Control=100.00%								
Subtle CD=0.00%								
Step 1								
ECog Planning	-1.30	0.53	6.03	1	.041	0.27	0.10, 0.77	.007
Constant	4.59	2.06	4.99	1	.026	98.61	-	-
Nagelkerke R^2=0.14								
Overall classification accuracy=66.20%								
Healthy Control=92.50%								
Subtle CD=24.00%								
Step 2								
ECog Planning	-1.65	0.58	8.02	1	.005	0.19	0.06, 0.60	.001
GDS total depressive symptoms	-0.18	0.09	3.78	1	.052	0.84	0.70, 1.00	.032
Constant	6.71	2.43	7.61	1	.006	820.180	-	-
Nagelkerke R^2=0.23								
Overall classification accuracy=76.90%								
Healthy Control=85.00%								
Subtle CD=64.00%								
Step 3								
ECog Planning	-1.74	0.61	8.11	1	.004	0.18	0.05, 0.58	.001
GDS total depressive symptoms	-0.33	0.12	7.34	1	.007	0.72	0.56, 0.91	.001
AMAS-E physiological anxiety	0.14	0.06	5.94	1	.015	1.15	1.03, 1.28	.007
Constant	1.63	3.11	0.28	1	0.60	5.11	-	-
Nagelkerke R^2=0.34								
Overall accuracy=78.50%								
Healthy Control=92.50%								
Subtle CD=56.00%								

Table 3.5 Power analyses: Sample size required at lower and upper power thresholds

Predictor	Source	OR	Sample Size: Power 0.40	Sample Size: Power 0.70
SCD (for Subtle CD)*	-	1.50	191	462
Subtle CD (for SCD)*	-	1.50	191	462
Age	Age (Balash et al., 2013)	1.01	79024	192042
(Male) Sex*	Male Sex (Balash et al., 2013)	0.70	255	618
Education	Education >16 years (Krell-Roesch et al., 2015)	1.45	227	550
TOPF	Education >16 years (Krell-Roesch et al., 2015)	1.45	227	550
Family w/Dementia	-	1.50	191	462
Psych Dx.*	-	1.50	191	462
MATS Word-finding	-	1.50	55	127
ECog Memory	ECog Memory: Frailty (Gifford et al., 2019)	1.81	30	65
ECog Planning	ECog Planning: Frailty (Gifford et al., 2019)	2.63	16	31
ECog Organization	ECog Organization: Frailty (Gifford et al., 2019)	2.39	18	36
ECog Divided Attn.	ECog Divided Attn.: Frailty (Gifford et al., 2019)	1.71	34	77
CCI	-	1.50	55	127
GDS	GDS (Balash et al., 2013)	1.32	109	258
UCLA Loneliness	-	1.50	55	127
AMAS-E WOS	Geriatric Anxiety Inventory: Excessive Worry (Diefenbach et al., 2014)	1.86	28	60
AMAS-E PHYS	Geriatric Anxiety Inventory: Excessive Worry (Diefenbach et al., 2014)	1.86	28	60
AMAS-E FEAR	Geriatric Anxiety Inventory: Excessive Worry (Diefenbach et al., 2014)	1.86	28	60
AMAS-E LIE	Geriatric Anxiety Inventory: Excessive Worry (Diefenbach et al., 2014)	1.86	28	60
AMAS-E GENERAL	Geriatric Anxiety Inventory: Overall Anxiety (Diefenbach et al., 2014)	2.02	23	49

* Dichotomous variables; OR: Odds ratio.

Chapter 4: Clarifying the connection between qualitative reports and potential cognitive risk factors in older adulthood

Introduction

In recent years, subjective cognitive decline (SCD) has garnered a great deal of clinical interest as a potential early stage indicator for dementia and other pathological cognitive decline. Older adults with SCD report self-perceived cognitive decline despite performing within expected limits on objective clinical-neuropsychological measures (Jessen et al., 2014). While cognitive complaints are common – even typical – among healthy older adults (Cooper et al., 2011; Jonker, Geerlings, & Schmand, 2000), there is persuasive evidence to suggest that SCD may prove a strong predictor of non-normative cognitive decline in at least a sub-sample of these individuals (Reisberg, Shulman, Torossian, Leng, & Zhu, 2010). The challenge, then, lies in discriminating complaints that are predictive of pathological cognitive decline from the normative age-related complaints and concerns of typical older adulthood. Accurate identification of which self-reported cognitive changes are clinically significant may be key to instituting early intervention before impairment occurs (Imtiaz, Tolppanen, Kivipelto, & Soininen, 2014; Smart et al., 2017).

Issues with Quantitative Measurement of SCD-Related Risk

Shortcomings of standardized cognitive-neuropsychological assessment. Classifying SCD and measuring its objective sequelae has proven problematic. Individuals with SCD perform within normal limits on objective cognitive tests by definition (Jessen et al., 2014). Nevertheless, numerous attempts have been made to identify SCD-specific cognitive profiles that are indicative of underlying neuropathology. These attempts have met with limited success. Individuals with SCD have occasionally been found to perform more poorly than healthy controls (without SCD) on cognitive screening measures (Stewart et al., 2001), as well as clinical tests of simple attention (Fortea et al., 2011), memory (Jessen et al., 2007), and executive functioning (Fonseca et al., 2015; Smart & Krawitz, 2015); however, these results have not been consistently replicated. This outcome is not entirely unexpected given the psychometric properties of standardized clinical-neuropsychological measures, which are optimized for detecting cognitive impairment significant enough to impact daily functioning. As a result, such tests are exceptional at identifying those with frank impairment but are relatively insensitive to incremental differences in normal-range, unimpaired performance. While such measures have proven invaluable for identifying clinical samples, they are ill-equipped to assess subclinical decrements as may be present in SCD.

Shortcomings of self-report measures. Given the inadequacy of standardized cognitive-neuropsychological measures, the determination of SCD has relied primarily on self-report measures. However, these have also suffered from issues of insensitivity, lack of specificity, and general lack of clinical consensus (Rabin et al., 2015). Much like standardized cognitive tests, the majority of self-report measures available are designed to detect blatant cognitive impairment in select domains (e.g., memory) amongst identified clinical populations such as persons with mild cognitive impairment (MCI) or dementia. Consequently, they may lack the requisite sensitivity or specificity to capture the full extent of SCD-related concerns and experiences. Other measures are designed to capture normative age-related cognitive complaints in the healthy older adult population, and as such may result in false positives with regard to classification of SCD (Rabin et al., 2015). Of particular relevance to SCD, few measures differentiate between the presence of *concern* about cognitive decline from the actual occurrence of cognitive complaints. That is, while many older adults may perceive cognitive complaints as part and parcel of normal aging, others may be very troubled by this decline and what it represents – persons who are now more likely to be classified as having SCD. Accordingly, self-report measures alone may lack sensitivity for discriminating normative age-related concerns from those suggestive of burgeoning pathology (Rabin et al., 2015).

The Case for a (Novel) Qualitative Approach

SCD as currently conceptualized is a fairly recent area of study, and the first-person subjective experience of persons with SCD remains largely unknown. Although numerous efforts have been and are being made to identify optimally sensitive measures and specific quantitative predictors of cognitive decline, it remains unclear whether these quantitative assessments truly reflect the full spectrum of concerns for those with SCD. As a result, important diagnostic information rooted in the subjective experience may be disregarded or overlooked. This need for documenting the first-person experience of persons with SCD has been explicitly acknowledged by researchers in the field (e.g., Buckley, Saling, Frommann, Wolfsgruber, & Wagner, 2015; Rabin et al., 2015). Qualitative approaches are not only ideal for theory building, in-depth description, and test construction, but may also parallel actual clinical interactions more closely than traditional "laboratory" methods. As frontline clinicians are likely to be presented with individuals' subjective accounts, identifying risk indicators within qualitative reports may be essential to efficient streaming of care.

The benefits of understanding the qualitative aspects of SCD are substantial; however, qualitative investigations of SCD have not been pursued with the same fervor as quantitative studies. While this may be due in part to clinicians' comfort and familiarity with post-positivist quantitative epistemologies, it is also true that qualitative methods alone – or at least as have been conducted – may be unable to immediately provide the clear diagnostic guidance sought by clinical researchers and practitioners. For instance, qualitative efforts to characterize SCD to date have relied heavily on phenomenological approaches (Buckley et al., 2015). Such approaches are uniquely well-suited for exploring first-hand experiences and identifying overarching experiential themes; however, they require "bracketing" of existing knowledge (e.g., approaching each interaction as a "blank slate"), which makes the accumulation and refinement of clinically-relevant information difficult (Creswell & Poth, 2017). The compiled results of these phenomenological studies provide excellent insight into patient impact but, due to the natural variance of interpretive outcomes, the necessity of disregarding previous findings, and the primary focus on patient experience rather than clinical practice, may be sub-optimal for developing concrete clinical applications.

Nevertheless, qualitative data may yet garner practical and useful clinical information. Where thematic data provided by interpretive approaches (e.g., phenomenology) may be difficult to translate directly into clinical practice, more concrete approaches based on the categorization and analysis of specific self-reported content may be more appropriate. More specifically, evaluation of the frequency of experience endorsement across various risk groups may provide an opportunity to evaluate the risk potential of commonly reported complaints in a rigorous and replicable fashion. By applying quantitative analytical methods to qualitative data, the information provided by patient self-reports may be most easily cross-validated with existing self-report measures, compared against cognitive-neuropsychological assessment data and, eventually, viably integrated into current screening and intake practices. Correspondingly, and as a first step, our chief objective in this study was to quantitatively determine the association between SCD, lower than expected cognitive performance (i.e., subtle cognitive decline; subtle CD), and endorsement of older adults' specific lived experiences of aging and cognitive change. We refrained from generating specific hypotheses due to the early and exploratory nature of this work. It is our hope that our results will serve as a foundation for the generation of meaningful hypotheses as this work is expanded.

Methods

Participants

Eligibility criteria and recruitment details are summarized in chapter 2.

Quantitative Sources of Data

Self-report measures. Participants completed self-report scales related to depression, anxiety, loneliness, and demographic factors to be used as covariates in our analyses. A complete list of administered self-report measures is provided in Table 3.1 and is summarized in full in chapter 3 of this book.

Neuropsychological assessment. Subtle CD (Edmonds, Delano-Wood, Galasko, Salmon, & Bondi, 2015) was determined by analyzing patterns of lower performance across a neuropsychological assessment battery designed to closely parallel the Uniform Data Set used in the large-scale ADNI study (Weintraub et al., 2018). The complete battery is outlined in Table 4.1 and summarized in full in chapter 2 of this book. Our revised criteria and operational definition for subtle CD in the current project is likewise summarized in chapter 2.

Qualitative Sources of Data

Semi-structured interview. Given our aim to parallel a clinical encounter and represent the types of disclosures likely to occur in those contexts, qualitative data was obtained via a directed content analysis approach (Hsieh & Shannon, 2005). A semi-structured interview schedule was created to address the areas typically explored during a clinical/neuropsychological intake interview. These items pertained to functioning within various cognitive domains, one's emotional functioning, and views around age-related change. Though the prepared interview items served as a foundation, deviations were permitted as necessary in response to participants' disclosures or preference. Further, specific topic areas were approached flexibly in the order and with the wording that made most sense within the context of the interaction. The semi-structured interview schedule is presented in the Table 4.A2 (Appendix).

Outcomes

Interview data were coded according to specific experiential content and similarity with other participants' accounts. As applicable, codes were grouped into hierarchical categories related to behavioural and cognitive domains, and overarching descriptive themes. F-values, p-values, and ηp^2 effect sizes are provided for the potential main and interacting effects of group (i.e., SCD, subtle CD) on total number of codes endorsed within a given category. p-values for covariate effects on total codes endorsed per category are also summarized.

Procedures

The study procedures were approved by the University of Victoria Human Research Ethics Board and all activities were conducted in accordance with the Declaration of Helsinki.

Qualitative interviews. Following telephone screening and consent procedures, participants completed a one-on-one semi-structured interview with the study's Principal Investigator (JIA) at a local academic institution. Participants were provided the opportunity to openly discuss their experiences of cognitive and related functional change/stability with age. Where necessary, participants were provided prompts to discuss the cognitive aspects of aging or to address specific neuropsychological domains. When cognitive declines were reported, participants were asked to elaborate on any related concerns, functional disruptions, compensatory strategies, and/or emotional responses. Interviews ranged from 30 minutes to one hour, depending on participants' responses and conversational flow. Interviews were audio-recorded with participants' consent. Field notes regarding interview content and observations were logged during and following each interview.

Transcription. Following completion of the interview, each audio recording was independently transcribed by two trained research assistants. Conflicts between files were reconciled by the Principal Investigator (JIA) prior to finalization of transcripts.

Member check. Telephone member checks were performed to ensure the validity of the ensuing thematic analysis. That is, several weeks following completion of an interview, participants were emailed a summary of points derived from their conversation with the Principal Investigator. Summaries delineated reported declines, gains, and stability across specific cognitive/functional domains. After reviewing their respective summary, participants arranged a follow-up telephone interview with the Principal Investigator. During telephone follow-up, participants were asked to correct any perceived inaccuracies in the summary, to elaborate on points where necessary, and provide any additional insights that may have occurred following the interview experience. Telephone interviews were also recorded and changes noted. Six participants made slight amendments to their initial reports during the member check: $n=3$ acknowledged greater concern or perceived changes while $n=3$ reported fewer. An additional $n=3$ reported that their summaries accurately depicted their experience at the time of the interview but that their degree of concern or challenge had since lessened due to external factors (e.g., the removal of an environmental stressor, treatment for depression).

Analyses

Content analysis. Initial coding and categorization of qualitative data was independently conducted by the Principal Investigator. Transcripts were reviewed thoroughly and qualitative experiences were coded inclusively. Coding was conducted via a constant comparative process such that previous transcripts were revisited as additional interview data became available (Fram, 2013). Each code was entered into a database and assigned a binary value to indicate whether it was endorsed or absent per participant. This was consistent with methods used previously by (Miebach, Wolfsgruber, Frommann, Buckley, & Wagner, 2018) in their study of cognitive complaint profiles. Codes endorsed by fewer than five participants were discarded from analysis. Codes endorsed by more than five participants were combined into superordinate categories and then larger descriptive themes.

Procedural rigour/trustworthiness. Qualitative rigour relies on the principle of "trustworthiness", which comprises credibility, transferability/generalizability, dependability, and confirmability (Lincoln & Guba, 1985). These aspects of trustworthiness will be discussed in order. Credibility in this study is considered relatively high given that statistical comparisons were applied to our qualitative data. Likewise, our cognitive domain categories were based on neuropsychological research and clinical convention, increasing the likelihood that the categorization of cognitive change experiences is objectively credible. To further support this, the categorization of reported cognitive change experiences to specific cognitive domains was checked for accuracy by an author (CMS) who is a clinical neuropsychologist. Our member check also ensured that our findings were credible in so far as they accurately reflected the felt experiences of our participants. As always, however, confidence in the credibility of this study is not complete. Our low *n* made it difficult to conduct meaningful analyses at the item level and may have undermined our power to detect objective differences in experiential endorsement at the category level as well.

Despite our relatively strong credibility, the transferability of our findings remains unclear. However, this may be tied to our specific sample rather than our data collection or analyses. Our sample of older adults were unique in that they were generally highly educated, were physically fit, previously worked in a professional capacity, and lived within a relatively high socioeconomic bracket. It is understood that, while our population was somewhat reflective of the local demographic, these characteristics are far from typical for other communities. Our sample may have been additionally selective given the (perceived) subject matter of the study as well. It was noted by several participants that their reasons for participating were that they believed themselves to be aging in an exemplary manner. Indeed, many claimed that they functioned better than the majority of their peers across a variety of cognitive and behavioural areas. Others shared that their peers with cognitive concerns were reticent to participant for fear of learning that they may have dementia. Together, this suggests that our sample was not only distinct due to their various demographic characteristics but may also have represented those who were particularly well-functioning. As such, our findings should be considered with caution when applying to older adults in different communities.

The dependability and credibility of our study equates with the quantitative notions of reliability and validity, respectively. Our findings were based on the data that was obtained without embellishment or undue interpretation. Cognitive domains were determined by clinical convention and neuropsychological research. Behavioural changes were determined according to the the degree of similarity between various compensatory strategies or lifestyle adjustments. These were clarified during the initial interviews as well as during the member check follow-ups. Participants were asked to clarify their experiences, the frequency of their experiences, their beliefs about the meaning of experiences, and the impact of endorsed experiences. Additional steps were taken by the Principal Investigator to ensure freedom from bias. Following each research encounter, the Principal Investigator engaged in reflexive journaling to make clearer their own responses to participants' and reported experiences. Note was also made of contextual factors and deviations from the semi-structured interview schedule. The only known threat to dependability over time is that the subject matter is subjective and that individuals' perceptions of their own strengths, weaknesses, and changes may shift over time. This was evident even within the short interval between the initial interviews and member check follow ups. Given the potential and inherent volatility of self-perceptions and comfort with disclosure, it is likely that participants' reports may differ from occasion to occasion. Nevertheless, our results are considered a credible and accurate representation of our sample's reported experiences at the time of the study.

Statistical comparison. All statistical analyses were performed using SPSS statistical software, Version 27. Chi-squared analyses and independent samples t-tests were conducted to examine the equivalence of group characteristics. Multivariate ANOVA (MANOVA) was conducted to determine the potential effect(s) of SCD and subtle CD on the mean endorsement of specific categories of qualitative experience. MANOVA analyses were only conducted for category-level data. Category mean scores served as ersatz subscale totals and were considered more robust than item-level data given our small sample size and the binary nature of coded content endorsement (Lezak, Howieson, Bigler, & Tranel, 2012). Covariables included in the MANOVA were participant age, sex, years of education, whether participants had a first-degree relative with dementia, whether participants held a historical or current psychiatric diagnosis, depressive symptomology (Geriatric Depression Scale; GDS), loneliness (UCLA Loneliness Scale), worry/oversensitivity (Adult Manifest Anxiety Scale; AMAS), physiological anxiety (AMAS), fear of aging (AMAS), response bias (AMAS), and total anxiety (AMAS). Granted the exploratory nature of this work, we felt the inclusion of multiple covariates to be justifiable. Post-hoc Bonferroni correction was employed for between-subjects effects to mitigate the inflation of family-wise error due to multiple comparisons. Independent samples Mann-Whitney U tests were performed instead for outcomes found to violate the assumptions of normality/homoscedasticity.

Results

Sample Characteristics

Demographic data and self-report outcomes for eligible participants are provided in Table 2 and are summarized in full in chapter 2 of this book.

Codes, Categories, and Themes

Commonly endorsed experiences were grouped across three nested levels: (1) coded content, (2) superordinate categories of coded content reflecting behavioural and cognitive domains, and (3) organizing themes related to overarching spheres of functioning. Coded content (1) reflected specific experiences commonly reported by participants. Following transcript review, coding, and extraction, a total n=38 individual coded experiences were identified. Exemplar quotes per content code are provided in Table 4.3. Next, secondary categories (2) were established. Content codes related to perceived cognitive decline (n=29 codes) were grouped according to common underlying cognitive domains. These cognitive categories comprised "Attention/Processing Decline", "Executive Function Decline", "Memory Decline", "Language Decline", and "Visuospatial Decline". Notably, codes related to simple attention, sustained attention, and processing speed and efficiency were grouped together in correspondence with common clinical frameworks (e.g., Lezak, Howieson, Bigler, & Tranel, 2012). Similarly, working memory, divided attention, selective attention, switching, and inhibition were categorized collectively as executive functions (e.g., Diamond, 2013). As an infrequently endorsed code, issues with navigation and/or orientation were singularly categorized under visuospatial processing. Although this code and category were barely represented in our sample, it was deemed important to categorize explicitly, as visuospatial processing is a commonly assessed cognitive domain and has been associated with early signs of cognitive decline in previous studies (Amariglio,

Townsend, Grodstein, Sperling, & Rentz, 2011). The consistent and accurate categorization of reported experiences into neuropsychological domains was checked by CMS, co-author and clinical neuropsychologist. Similar to behavioural categories, a "Total Decline" category was defined to summarize the total number of endorsements across all other cognitive change categories. Content codes related to behavioural changes (n=9 codes) were grouped according to similarity of compensatory response or functional aim. Behavioural categories comprised "Anticipating (Cognitive/Functional) Decline", "Reducing Cognitive Load", "Organizing (one's) Environment", and "Increasing Exposure (to stimuli)". An additional "Total Strategies" category was generated to reflect the total number of endorsed codes across all behavioural categories. Finally, identified categories were divided into two major themes (3) alluded to above, "Cognitive Change" and "Behavioural Change" for organizational ease. A complete summary of content codes per category and theme is provided in Table 4.4.

Effects of SCD and Subtle CD on Qualitative Experience Endorsement

Levene's test indicated that that several experiential category outcomes violated the assumption of homoscedasticity; namely, Language Decline (p=.026), Visuospatial Processing Decline (p=.009), Anticipating Decline (p=.002), Increasing Exposure (p<.000), and Total Compensatory Strategies (p=.023). Accordingly, SCD and subtle CD group effects on these variables were analyzed via independent samples Mann-Whitney U tests. All remaining dependent variables demonstrated normally distributed data, correlated well, and were entered into MANOVA analyses.

Omnibus effects of SCD and subtle CD.

Frequency of code endorsement and mean number of codes endorsed within a given category are presented by group in Table 4.5. Significance values (p-values) and associated effect size estimates of SCD and subtle CD between-group effects are provided in Table 4.6. Few significant covariate effects were found to impact the endorsement of behavioural changes (Theme 2 categories) and none were found to impact the endorsement of cognitive changes (Theme 2 categories). A complete summary of covariate effects (p-values) per category and themes is presented in Table A.41 (Appendix).

MANOVA multivariate tests indicated no significant omnibus effects of SCD (Wilks' λ=.729, p=.181) or subtle CD (Wilks' λ=.781, p=.369) on qualitative experience endorsement. Likewise, no significant SCD x subtle CD interaction effect was found (Wilks' λ=.881, p=.853). Nevertheless, owing to our underpowered analyses due to our low n and the exploratory nature of this study, we felt further investigation into between-subject effects was still warranted.

Between-subject effects of SCD and subtle CD on category-level outcomes.

Theme 1: Cognitive Change. MANOVA between-subject analyses found participants with SCD to endorse significantly more Executive Functioning Decline codes (M=3.73, SD=1.45) compared to those who were unconcerned (M=2.05, SD=1.38; p<.010, ηp^2=.128). The presence of SCD was also associated with a higher number of reported cognitive changes overall (M=8.18, SD=2.56) versus unconcerned participants (M=5.65, SD=2.70; p=.040, ηp^2=.083), though this was likely driven by the primary effect on Executive Function Decline endorsement. In contrast with this SCD effect, subtle CD appeared to suppress the endorsement of executive functioning changes instead (M=2.16, SD=1.28) relative to healthy controls (M=2.90, SD=1.74; p<.023, ηp^2=.101). No SCD X subtle CD interaction was identified. Mann-Whitney U test found no significant effect of SCD or subtle CD on Language Decline or Visuospatial Processing Decline.

Theme 2: Behavioural Change. Mann-Whitney U test results indicated that those who endorsed SCD reported significantly more Increasing Exposure experiences/strategies (M=0.50,

SD=.060) than unconcerned individuals (M=0.14, SD=0.35; p=.005). A trending effect of SCD group on Anticipating Decline was also found (p=.054), whereby individuals who endorsed SCD (M=0.32, SD=0.57) were more likely to prepare for the possibility of dementia than unconcerned individuals (M=0.09, SD=0.29). As a result, the SCD group was found to endorse a greater number of behavioural changes overall (M=2.46, SD=1.30) relative to those without SCD (M=1.19, SD=0.88; p<.000). No other main or interaction effects of SCD or subtle CD on Theme 2 content were found.

Trending item-level effects. Exploratory secondary analysis (MANOVA) was conducted at the item-level of data to investigate any potential areas for greater emphasis in future work (i.e., coded content). The outcomes of these analyses were not presented as primary results given our low n, the large number of potential dependent variables (i.e., content codes), and the consequent statistical volatility of the findings. Nevertheless, we feel it pertinent to present these outcomes here to provide context for future work. We do so with the caveat that these outcomes may well be spurious and that they should be considered with appropriate caution. See Table 4.5 for a summary of item endorsement frequency.

With regard to Theme 1 coded content, we found subtle CD to have an effect on the endorsement of activity derailment; however, this effect was found to be non-significant following post-hoc analysis (χ^2=3.48, p=.062). SCD was not found to have any independent effect on specific coded content; however, several SCD x subtle CD interaction effects were indicated. A significant interaction effect was found to influence the endorsement of increased attentional effort (p=.013, ηp^2=.120). Healthy controls with SCD were significantly more likely to endorse increased attentional effort versus unconcerned controls (χ^2=6.71, p=.010). In contrast, those with concurrent subtle CD and SCD were significantly *less* inclined to report the same (χ^2=7.11, p=.008). In other words, SCD alone increased endorsement of attentional effort but, when paired with subtle CD, the presence of SCD led to a reduction in endorsement. Inversely, a more expected interaction effect was found to impact the endorsement of several other codes. Chi square analysis revealed that participants with subtle CD and SCD were more likely to endorse losing track of conversational topic compared to healthy controls with SCD (χ^2=3.87, p=.049). Similarly, both memory for conversations and sequencing were significantly more likely to be endorsed by those with SCD and subtle CD compared to healthy controls with SCD (χ^2=5.02, p=.025) or unconcerned individuals with subtle CD (χ^2=6.06, p=.014).

With regard to Theme 2 coded content, SCD and subtle CD both demonstrated independent effects on the endorsement of repetition and rehearsal; however, following post-hoc χ^2 analysis, only the SCD effect remained viable. Individuals endorsing SCD were significantly more likely to report an increase in mental rehearsal and repetition to maintain information in working memory compared to those without SCD (χ^2=6.90, p=.009).

Discussion

The goal of this study was to determine which, if any, self-reported experiences of aging and cognition related to the potential prodromal dementia risk factors of SCD and subtle CD. Due to a small sample size and considerable variability in individual item endorsement, statistical analyses were conducted at the category-level only. Overall, SCD was found to exert a more robust influence on the endorsement of specific categories of experience than subtle CD.

Findings

Theme 1: Cognitive Changes. With regard to self-perceived cognitive declines, both SCD and subtle CD exerted a significant independent influence on cognitive change category endorsement. More interestingly, both SCD and subtle CD were uniquely associated with the endorsement of a single category of perceived cognitive change: Executive Function Decline. The implication of executive functioning/fluid reasoning change is not particularly surprising given that these require the greatest number of cognitive resources and are the very domains known to degrade most with age (Harada et al., 2013; Murman, 2015). For instance, tracking a developing conversation while formulating pertinent responses in real time requires a high degree of online processing. Keeping up with conversation may entail working memory (e.g., remembering what was said and using it to inform one's response), divided attention (e.g., attending to incoming information while formulating and a delivering a response at the appropriate time), and inhibitory control (e.g., maintaining focus despite internal and external distractors or competing motivations) demands. What is notable, however, is that SCD and subtle CD appear to exert opposing effects on Executive Function Decline endorsement. Where those with SCD were more likely to endorse executive function decrements than those without, individuals with subtle (objective) cognitive decline were counterintuitively *less* inclined to endorse the same compared to healthy controls. This divergence suggests that SCD and subtle CD may reflect unique aspects of the cognitive aging experience rather than conferring multiplicative risk as might otherwise be expected given their individual identification as risk factors for objective cognitive decline in previous work (Edmonds et al., 2015; Jessen et al., 2014).

While it is unclear exactly what may underlie this difference in effect, there are several speculative explanations. An initial possibility is that those with subtle CD may potentially experience a more advanced degree of cognitive decline than those with SCD. If so, (some of) those with subtle CD may present with a degree of anosognosia (e.g., unawareness of one's own abilities and deficits). This would serve to preferentially suppress reports of cognitive decline in those with subtle CD but not those with SCD alone. However, as attractive as this explanation may be, the likelihood that our participants experienced neuropathological decline advanced enough to elicit anosognosia is low. Each performed well upon cognitive screening and soundly within normal limits on more advanced neuropsychological tests. Further, each of our participants continued to function well in their daily lives. A more viable alternative may be that those with SCD who have experienced few concrete changes in their ability may seek validation of their concerns, while those with subtle CD who have been confronted with more apparent declines may be less inclined to report them lest the possibility of neurodegeneration is reinforced. While this case for defensive denial is also intriguing, it is difficult to evaluate given our data. If true, one might expect those with subtle CD to be less inclined to endorse SCD. We did not find any significant difference in SCD endorsement between healthy controls and those with subtle CD though it is possible that our n was too low and our analyses too underpowered to detect any such effect.

Theme 2: Behavioural Changes. With regard to compensatory strategies and behavioural changes, older adults with SCD endorsed a greater number of change experiences overall compared to unconcerned individuals. Closer analysis revealed that this group difference was driven primarily by an SCD-specific increase in behaviours aimed at increasing the amount of exposure to information/stimuli in order to effectively maintain it in working memory (e.g., rehearsing information in mind). The greater endorsement of compensatory strategies overall was expected for those with SCD, however, the exclusivity of the effect on Increasing Exposure (i.e., strategies related to repetition, rehearsal, and reviewing information) was not anticipated. Given the selectivity of this effect, some degree of objective cognitive decline in the areas of working memory/executive functioning may be suspected. This, of course, would remain consistent with our Theme 1 findings. But what is unique to Increasing Exposure that leads it to be endorsed while other strategies are not?

One possibility may be that the characteristics of Increasing Exposure strategies cause them to be more easily undertaken or openly reported versus other strategies. Increasing Exposure strategies may simply be less burdensome than more overt strategies, like reorganizing one's physical space or avoiding certain tasks. Moreover, Increasing Exposure strategies may also be less threatening for those who are already concerned about the potential of dementia (e.g., those with subtle CD). Where more obvious strategies may unquestionably signal to an individual that their abilities have changed, the more habitual strategies of the Increasing Exposure category may obviate the deliberate identification of deficits or purposeful adjustment of daily routines. Further, given the internalized – even invisible – nature of some Increasing Exposure strategies (e.g., mentally rehearsing information), individuals may be able to engage in these behaviours more surreptitiously. This may be particularly valuable in cases where individuals fear stigma or judgment from others related to their perceived cognitive changes (e.g., Corner & Bond, 2004). In other words, Increasing Exposure strategies may be more accessible and, perhaps, even more attractive to individuals managing (perceived) cognitive changes.

Another contributing factor to the salience of Increasing Exposure compensatory strategies for those with SCD may be the characteristics of the underlying target abilities of working memory, attentional control, and broad executive functioning. Each of these abilities may broadly fall under the banner of fluid reasoning abilities (Lezak et al., 2012). Fluid reasoning abilities are known to decrease with age due to cortical atrophy in areas related to executive functioning, such as the dorsolateral prefrontal cortex, and degradation in more widely distributed processing networks (Glisky, 2007; Harada, Natelson Love, & Triebel, 2013; Murman, 2015). Chief among these affected abilities are working memory, processing speed, and inhibitory control (Glisky, 2007; McNab et al., 2015; Salthouse, Mitchell, Skovronek, & Babcock, 1989). *In situ*, these age-related decrements manifest as decreased resistance to distraction, slower and less efficient encoding of information, and increased effort to maintain and manipulate information in one's mind. Consequently, it may well be that Increasing Exposure strategies are more commonly undertaken due to the regularity and pervasiveness of the executive functioning/working memory challenges they address.

Finally, it is likely that the characteristics of those with SCD and their concerns may contribute to the endorsement of Increasing Exposure strategies specifically. Where episodic memory decrements are often expected to occur with age, these working memory and complex attentional challenges may be less anticipated by older adults and, consequently, may be experienced as more foreign and threatening than otherwise. This may be even more so for those who historically counted these abilities amongst their greatest strengths (e.g., the academics and administrators comprising our sample). These unexpected – and typically unwelcomed – changes may collaborate to undermine older adults' confidence in their cognitive abilities, convince them that specific cognitive tasks necessarily require management, and elicit concerns about potential loss of independence (Hill et al., 2016). In response, high-functioning older adults may be prone to habitually engaging in cognitive strategies to maintain a consistent degree of productivity while simultaneously staving off the suggestion of incompetence. Indeed, returning to an earlier point, it is likely no coincidence that SCD increased the performance of an internal (i.e., covert) strategy but had no impact on more outwardly apparent behavioural changes. This may also align with our interpretation of the conflicting SCD and subtle CD effects on Executive Functioning Decline (Theme 1). Where those with SCD alone may be driven to compensate and report their challenges/adjustments, those who suspect more pronounced decrements (i.e., subtle CD) may emphasize warding against scrutiny and negative judgment instead. As a result those with subtle CD may be reticent to acknowledge their declines by adjusting their habits and/or openly reporting that they have done so.

Suggestive item-level endorsement. Content-level review revealed that, of the various content codes loading onto fluid reasoning, the impacted items were those with the most direct, concrete, and (outwardly) apparent impact on socialization and daily functioning. Although decline in other fluid reasoning-contingent abilities was commonly reported by our sample (e.g., processing speed decrements), the endorsement of SCD only increased significantly when individuals experienced objective decline in executive areas with clear behavioural consequences. This suggests that SCD may best reflect the downstream ecological effects of objective decline in processing speed, updating/working memory, planning and inhibitory control. In other words, SCD may be an indicator of observed executive functioning decrements rather than memory impairment as it has most often been interpreted.

Situating within the qualitative literature. As mentioned previously, few qualitative studies on SCD have been conducted. Those that have been conducted have primarily utilized a phenomenological approach (e.g., Buckley et al., 2015) that is appropriate for describing broad experiential themes among comparable populations but falls short as a means for identifying specific items that may prove clinically significant. Thus, there is little literature against which to compare our found effects against. Nevertheless, there are several studies that may provide some degree of convergent evidence to support the validity of our item-level findings.

As part of the large-scale Nurse's Health Study, Amariglio et al. (Amariglio et al., 2011) conducted a survey of the specific subjective memory complaints reported by 16,960 older women with or without cognitive impairment. Rather than the open-ended method used in the current study, Amariglio and coworkers asked participants to indicate whether any of seven specific cognitive complaints applied to them. They found that endorsement of two complaints in particular predicted participants' cognitive status: difficulty keeping up with conversation and difficulties with orientation/navigation. Although their study focused exclusively on item-level (i.e., coded content) analysis, some of Amariglio et al.'s findings align well with our own. Tracking a developing conversation while formulating pertinent responses in real time requires a high degree of online processing and executive functioning. Keeping up with conversation may entail working memory (e.g., remembering what was said and using it to inform one's response), divided attention (e.g., attending to incoming information while formulating and delivering a response at the appropriate time), and inhibitory control (e.g., maintaining focus despite internal and external distractors or competing motivations) demands. In the midst of discourse, efficiently encoding the content to memory requires exponentially more cognitive resources. Thus, while our category-level finding that Executive Function Decline is associated with both SCD and subtle CD corresponds broadly with Amariglio et al.'s results, our trending item-level effects are even more consistent with their findings.

While difficulties keeping up with conversations aligns with our trending item-level results, orientation/navigation challenges do not. Given that Amariglio et al.'s (2011) cognitively impaired sample was significantly more compromised than our subtle CD sample, however, this is not surprising. It is quite possible that difficulties keeping up with conversation may present earlier in the cognitive decline trajectory and/or may be more sensitive to the subtle disruptions in cognitive functioning expected to occur in advance of pathological decline. Alternatively, it is equally possible that challenges with keeping up with conversation may simply be encountered more regularly than navigation challenges as older adults begin to lessen their involvement with driving. Yet another possibility may be that conversational challenges are more readily disclosed than navigation issues, as many older adult participants acknowledged visuospatial deficits as troubling and a potential marker of dementia. Even without the possibility of dementia, several participants shared that the loss of their driver's license would be experienced as catastrophic for them. As a result, it is probable that some may have censored their reports around this domain specifically. Whatever the reason for this divergence, the reinforcement of difficulties keeping up with conversation as a sensitive indicator of potential cognitive pathology is heartening.

Another, more recent study by Miebach et al. (2018) explored the lived experiences of adults with cognitive complaints in comparison to those with major depressive disorder and healthy controls. In their study, Miebach et al. conducted a semi-structured interview more closely aligned with the methods used in the current study. Given that the focus of their study was not to identify specific concerns or experiences of change, few of their outcomes related to these subjects at all. However, they did note that individuals with cognitive concerns demonstrated distractible speech significantly more than healthy controls during their interviews. This was operationalized as researcher-observed tangentiality, losing track of the topic at hand, and losing track of one's train of thought. While not entirely aligned with our findings, the features of distractible speech do overlap somewhat with our trending item-level finding that concerned (SCD) older adults with subtle CD may demonstrate higher endorsement of difficulties keeping up with conversation and the suggestion of executive functioning deficits.

Taken as a whole, these studies appear to provide some convergent evidence for the (subtle) disruption of executive functioning abilities in those who have cognitive complaints and, potentially, who may have incipient cognitive pathology. Further, these disruptions may manifest most readily to individuals and others in social/conversational contexts. With that said, it should be acknowledged that neither of these studies investigated SCD (e.g., concerned) populations *per se*, but rather those with cognitive complaints. However, given that those with SCD are considered to be at particularly high risk of developing pathological cognitive decline relative to those with complaints alone (Jessen et al., 2020), these convergent findings remain intriguing.

Clinical Implications

As the primary impetus behind this work was to help determine which self-reported cognitive and behavioural change experiences may provide the most utility for early dementia risk screening, the results present several important considerations for clinical practice and research. Foremost, our findings broadly support those of Amariglio et al. (2011) and Miebach et al. (2018) in that executive functioning decrements – and not episodic memory impairments – appear to be most associated with subtle and potentially early-stage cognitive decline. While this is somewhat intuitive given that executive functions are known to rely on distributed and synchronized neural networks which are particularly prone to disruption by insult or other pathology (Elliott, 2003; Rabinovici, Stephens, & Possin, 2015), this finding still conflicts with the majority of the SCD literature which remains focused on episodic memory as a primary index of cognitive (dys)function.

Several reasons may underlie this memory-centric view of SCD and dementia risk. For one, SCD and its progenitors (e.g., subjective memory complaints, cognitive concerns) were initially identified in memory clinical samples for the express purpose of identifying Alzheimer's-type pathology in that group. Given that these individuals presented to clinic with memory concerns specifically and that episodic memory decline is essentially pathognomonic of Alzheimer's dementia, it is understandable that memory was a chief concern for clinicians. In light of this historical foundation, the course of investigation into early cognitive risk factors for dementia has been slow to include other cognitive domains. Another reason why executive functioning may be under-represented in the current SCD literature is that the majority of studies continue to be based on clinical populations and episodic memory declines may be more immediately apparent and troubling for older adults. It is possible that, due to the lay public's association of memory impairment with dementia and the concreteness of memory slips, these are the symptoms most likely to elicit medical help-seeking behaviour. On the other hand, disruptions in executive functioning may be less apparent, less concrete, and less immediately threatening for older adults due to the lack of "buzz" around such cognitive changes. Taking this further, the concreteness of episodic memory changes may be simpler for clinicians and researchers to decipher as well. As mentioned previously, fluid reasoning and executive functioning decrements are expected to occur with age (McNab et al., 2015), making it challenging to parse "risky" executive changes from normative declines. For these reasons among others, executive functioning declines have been somewhat overshadowed by more explicit cognitive changes in the SCD literature, despite growing evidence suggesting that executive functioning is potentially as or even more sensitive to sub-clinical neuropathological disruption (Baudic et al., 2006).

The primary import of our findings, then, is that they indicate specific self-reported cognitive changes that may prove useful for early screening of dementia risk. Executive functioning declines, potentially in the form of self-reported challenges keeping up with conversation, encoding and recalling the details of past conversations, and inefficient planning and sequencing of daily activities, may suggest some degree of cognitive vulnerability and may manifest long before the more advanced pathological symptoms of episodic memory impairment and visuospatial deficits. Likewise, clinicians may observe challenges with distractible speech as outlined by Miebach et al. (2018). Although this was not assessed in the current study, it remains consistent with developing executive attention and inhibition deficits and may warrant attention during intake and screening procedures.

An additional benefit of our findings is that the change experiences endorsed by our ostensibly highest risk participants (i.e., those with SCD and subtle CD) were not those typically associated with incipient dementia or cognitive pathology. It has been noted previously that older adults who suspect that they are at risk of developing a cognitive pathology may be prone to under-reporting cognitive symptoms or otherwise attempting to distance themselves from the possibility of receiving a diagnosis (Beard & Neary, 2013). Community-based older adult samples may demonstrate similar tendencies. For instance, none of the participants in the current study had sought formal medical assessment and few reported researching their experiences independently (e.g., on the internet), regardless of their degree of concern. It is also possible that more commonly endorsed cognitive concerns, like memory failures, may have been under-reported by those seeking to distance themselves from any suggestion of Alzheimer's disease or dementia. Where under-reporting of symptoms explicitly related to dementia risk (e.g., memory failures) is a concern, conversationally querying concrete aspects of aging and daily functioning as a matter of routine may allow clinicians to bypass potential patient defensiveness without eliciting the existential threat posed by the possibility of dementia outright.

Limitations and Future Recommendations

Given the particularities of our sample, several qualifications are warranted. Aside from the sample size limitations reported in chapter 2, the specific occupational history, setting, and motivation of our participants may colour the generalizability of our findings. The majority of our sample were previous academics and professionals. Many explicitly voiced their belief that their cognitive abilities were superior to others their age and alluded to being motivated to participate because they believed they were aging in exemplary fashion. Indeed, many of our participants did perform in the high average – superior range on objective neuropsychological assessment. In light of their high cognitive reserve and baseline ability/functioning, it is quite possible that our findings and our sample at large may be more characteristic of those with a certain degree of cognitive resiliency. Related, given that our participants were accustomed to being viewed as capable and cognitively superior to others in many cases, they may have been more reticent to share details of perceived cognitive decline openly. This defensive responding may have disproportionately suppressed the report of cognitive changes commonly associated with dementia risk (e.g., episodic memory slips) over others. It is possible that participant disclosure may also have been suppressed somewhat by the academic setting of the study and/or the relative youth of the Principal Investigator. Indeed, it was observed that many participants adopted a pseudo-mentorship role throughout the data collection process despite being the subjects of the study.

Another notable feature of our sample that may have compounded this tendency toward guardedness may have been the disproportionately high number of female participants vs. male participants (78.5%). The women in our sample were unique in that they represented female professionals who were active during a time when the professional and academic environments were altogether inhospitable for women. Many would have entered the workforce during the crest of the second-wave of the feminist movement and would have been seen as iconoclasts. Indeed, many of our participants attested to this directly. As a result of their experiences with overcoming institutional obstacles and cultural rebuke (i.e., cultures of sexism, such as reduced opportunities for advancement due to sex/gender, etc.), our sample of professional women may have developed personas characterized by invulnerability and unquestionable competence (Friedman & Yorio,

2006; Shaw & Hoeber, 2003). Related, they may have been somewhat biased toward demonstrating/disclosing resilience, and defending against any suggestion of vulnerability. This tendency may have been exaggerated further in the study setting, given that conversations focused on what may have equated to changes in core aspects of identity (e.g., competence, intelligence). The interacting contextual factors of being retired, female, professional, participating in a study about cognitive change, being interviewed in an academic setting, and being evaluated by a young male researcher may all have served to decrease our participants' openness to disclosing potential vulnerabilities.

Other limitations relate more to the study design. To ensure that participants were not objectively cognitively impaired, neuropsychological testing was conducted in advance of qualitative interviews. While this was beneficial for confirming the eligibility and validity of our sample before the additional investment of time and study resources, participant's experiences during testing may have influenced their openness and disclosed experiences during interview. Although participants were not provided feedback regarding their cognitive test performance, some were convinced that they had "failed" or that they would have performed "better" several years ago. These beliefs often persisted even when reminded that actual test performance was mutually exclusive from one's felt sense of achievement. Thus, as a result of their testing experiences, participants may have evaluated their cognitive abilities differently or may have been more vigilant for cognitive challenges in advance of their qualitative interviews. A final design caveat pertains more broadly to qualitative methods in general. It is acknowledged that, as the interviewer and chief interpreter of collected data, the Principal Investigator's contribution to the collected data is not zero. The dynamic between the interviewer and interviewee likely influenced the type and amount of data collected, just as the Principal Investigators perspective would have shaped the specific content coding. With that said, efforts were made to mitigate the degree of researcher impact by conducting member checks to ensure fidelity to participant experience, parallel transcription to ensure accurate recording, and collaborative categorization of content codes to ensure inter-rater reliability.

Future iterations of this work would benefit from a larger and more ethnically, socioeconomically, educationally, and sexually diverse sample. Longitudinal designs applying a similar methodology across various time points may help to discern which specific experiences may be most predictive of decline, as well as determine the chronology of developing self-perceived cognitive changes. Alternatively, additional cross-sectional studies investigating endorsed cognitive and behavioural change experiences among healthy controls, those with subtle CD, and those with objective cognitive decline (e.g., mild cognitive impairment) may approximate this same developmental trajectory. Similar to chapter 2, direct comparison of clinical and community-based samples with SCD would also help to clarify which experiences may be more readily endorsed by older adults in various settings, with various degrees of cognitive concern, and with varying degrees of openness to medical intervention.

Conclusions

Our findings indicate that those demonstrating sub-clinical cognitive declines and reporting concern about the potential of developing dementia may be more likely to report decrements in functional and social activities reliant on executive functions, such as working memory, inhibitory control, and divided attention. Those endorsing concerns who have not experienced functional disruptions, are more likely to report attentional tasks as requiring effort. Concern was also linked to a tendency toward mental rehearsal and review of material in order to compensate for perceived decrements in working memory and attention, regardless of objective ability. Taken together with convergent evidence, these results suggest that executive functioning – and not memory – decrements may be the earliest indications of potential cognitive vulnerability. The inclusion of concrete items related to conversational ability, memory for conversations, sequencing, and distractibility in routine cognitive screening measures/practices may be advantageous for early detection of those at increased risk of eventual dementia; however, their utility as screening items would require a greater degree of study within the context of a larger-scale longitudinal investigation.

Funding

This work was supported by the Alzheimer Society of Canada (Dr. & Mrs. Albert Spatz Award, 18-29) and the Lou-Poy family via the University of Victoria Institute on Aging and Lifelong Health (Alice Lou-Poy Graduate Scholarship).

References

Amariglio, R. E., Townsend, M. K., Grodstein, F., Sperling, R. A., & Rentz, D. M. (2011).

Specific subjective memory complaints in older persons may indicate poor cognitive

function. *Journal of the American Geriatrics Society, 59*(9), 1612–1617.

https://doi.org/10.1111/j.1532-5415.2011.03543.x

Baudic, S., Barba, G. D., Thibaudet, M. C., Smagghe, A., Remy, P., & Traykov, L. (2006).

Executive function deficits in early Alzheimer's disease and their relations with episodic

memory. *Archives of Clinical Neuropsychology, 21*(1), 15–21.

https://doi.org/10.1016/j.acn.2005.07.002

Beard, R. L., & Neary, T. M. (2013). Making sense of nonsense: Experiences of mild cognitive

impairment. *Sociology of Health & Illness, 35*(1), 130–146. https://doi.org/10.1111/j.1467-

9566.2012.01481.x

Buckley, R. F., Saling, M. M., Frommann, I., Wolfsgruber, S., & Wagner, M. (2015). Subjective

cognitive decline from a phenomenological perspective: A review of the qualitative

literature. *Journal of Alzheimer's Disease, 48*(Suppl 1), S125–S140.

https://doi.org/10.3233/JAD-150095

Cooper, C., Bebbington, P., Lindesay, J., Meltzer, H., McManus, S., Jenkins, R., & Livingston,

G. (2011). The meaning of reporting forgetfulness: A cross-sectional study of adults in the

English 2007 Adult Psychiatric Morbidity Survey. *Age and Ageing, 40*(6), 711–717.

https://doi.org/10.1093/ageing/afr121

Corner, L., & Bond, J. (2004). Being at risk of dementia: Fears and anxieties of older adults.

Nursing Older People, 18(2), 143–155. https://doi.org/10.7748/nop.16.5.8.s9

Creswell, J. W., & Poth, C. N. (2017). *Qualitative Inquiry and Research Design. Choosing*

Among Five Approaches. Thousand Oaks, CA: SAGE.

Diamond, A. (2013). Executive functions. *Annual Review of Psychology, 64*, 135–168.

https://doi.org/10.1146/annurev-psych-113011-143750

Edmonds, E. C., Delano-Wood, L., Galasko, D. R., Salmon, D. P., & Bondi, M. W. (2015).

Subtle cognitive decline and biomarker staging in preclinical Alzheimer's disease. *Journal*

of Alzheimer's Disease, 47(1), 231–242. https://doi.org/10.3233/JAD-150128

Elliott, R. (2003). Executive functions and their disorders: Imaging in clinical neuroscience.

British Medical Bulletin, 65(1), 49–59. https://doi.org/10.1093/bmb/65.1.49

Fonseca, J. A. S., Ducksbury, R., Rodda, J., Whitfield, T., Nagaraj, C., Suresh, K., … Walker, Z.

(2015). Factors that predict cognitive decline in patients with subjective cognitive

impairment. *International Psychogeriatrics/IPA*, *27*(10), 1671–1677.

https://doi.org/10.1017/S1041610215000356

Fortea, J., Sala-Llonch, R., Bartrés-Faz, D., Lladó, A., Solé-Padullés, C., Bosch, B., … Rami, L.

(2011). Cognitively preserved subjects with transitional cerebrospinal fluid β-amyloid 1-42

values have thicker cortex in Alzheimer's disease vulnerable areas. *Biological Psychiatry*,

70(2), 183–190. https://doi.org/10.1016/j.biopsych.2011.02.017

Fram, S. M. (2013). The constant comparative analysis method outside of grounded theory.

Qualitative Report, 18(1), 1–25.

Friedman, C., & Yorio, K. (2006). *The girl's guide to being a boss (without being a bitch):*

Valuable lessons, smart suggestions, and true stories for succeeding as the chick-in-charge.

New York, NY: Morgan Road Books.

Glisky, E. L. (2007). Changes in cognitive function in human aging. In D. R. Riddle (Ed.), *Brain*

aging: Models, methods, and mechanisms. Boca Raton, FL, USA: CRC Press/Taylor &

Francis.

Harada, C. N., Natelson Love, M. C., & Triebel, K. L. (2013). Normal cognitive aging. *Clinics in Geriatric Medicine, 29*(4), 737–752. https://doi.org/10.1016/j.cger.2013.07.002

Hill, N. L., Mogle, J., Wion, R., Munoz, E., DePasquale, N., Yevchak, A. M., & Parisi, J. M. (2016). Subjective cognitive impairment and affective symptoms: A systematic review. *Gerontologist, 56*(6), e109–e127. https://doi.org/10.1093/geront/gnw091

Hsieh, H.-F., & Shannon, S. E. (2005). Three approaches to qualitative content analysis. *Qualitative Health Research, 15*(9), 1277–1288.

Imtiaz, B., Tolppanen, A. M., Kivipelto, M., & Soininen, H. (2014). Future directions in Alzheimer's disease from risk factors to prevention. *Biochemical Pharmacology.* https://doi.org/10.1016/j.bcp.2014.01.003

Jessen, F., Amariglio, R. E., Buckley, R. F., van der Flier, W. M., Han, Y., Molinuevo, J. L., … Wagner, M. (2020). The characterisation of subjective cognitive decline. *The Lancet Neurology, 19*(3), 271–278. https://doi.org/10.1016/S1474-4422(19)30368-0

Jessen, F., Amariglio, R. E., Van Boxtel, M., Breteler, M., Ceccaldi, M., Chételat, G., … Wagner, M. (2014). A conceptual framework for research on subjective cognitive decline in preclinical Alzheimer's disease. *Alzheimer's and Dementia, 10*(6), 844–852. https://doi.org/10.1016/j.jalz.2014.01.001

Jessen, F., Wiese, B., Cvetanovska, G., Fuchs, A., Kaduszkiewicz, H., Kölsch, H., … Bickel, H. (2007). Patterns of subjective memory impairment in the elderly: Association with memory performance. *Psychological Medicine, 37*(12), 1753–1762. https://doi.org/10.1017/S0033291707001122

Jonker, C., Geerlings, M. I., & Schmand, B. (2000). Are memory complaints predictive for dementia? A review of clinical and population-based studies. *International Journal of Geriatric Psychiatry*, *15*(11), 983–991. https://doi.org/10.1002/1099-1166(200011)15:11<983::aid-gps238>3.0.co;2-5

Lezak, M. D., Howieson, D. B., Bigler, E. D., & Tranel, D. (2012). *Neuropsychological assessment, fifth edition*. New York, NY: Oxford University Press.

Lincoln, Y. S., & Guba, E. G. (1985). *Naturalistic inquiry*. Newbury Park, CA, USA: Sage.

McNab, F., Zeidman, P., Rutledge, R. B., Smittenaar, P., Brown, H. R., Adams, R. A., & Dolan, R. J. (2015). Age-related changes in working memory and the ability to ignore distraction. *Proceedings of the National Academy of Sciences of the United States of America, 112*(20), 6515–6518. https://doi.org/10.1073/pnas.1504162112

Miebach, L., Wolfsgruber, S., Frommann, I., Buckley, R., & Wagner, M. (2018). Different cognitive complaint profiles in memory clinic and depressive patients. *American Journal of Geriatric Psychiatry*, *26*(4), 463–475. https://doi.org/10.1016/j.jagp.2017.10.018

Murman, D. L. (2015). The Impact of Age on Cognition. *Seminars in Hearing, 36*(3), 111–121. https://doi.org/10.1055/s-0035-1555115

Rabin, L. A., Smart, C. M., Crane, P. K., Amariglio, R. E., Berman, L. M., Boada, M., … Sikkes, S. A. M. (2015). Subjective cognitive decline in older adults: An overview of self-report measures used across 19 international research studies. *Journal of Alzheimer's Disease*, *48*(S1), S63–S86. https://doi.org/10.3233/JAD-150154

Rabinovici, G. D., Stephens, M. L., & Possin, K. L. (2015). Executive dysfunction. *Continuum: Lifelong Learning in Neurology, 21*(3), 649–659.

Reisberg, B., Shulman, M. B., Torossian, C., Leng, L., & Zhu, W. (2010). Outcome over seven years of healthy adults with and without subjective cognitive impairment. *Neuropsychology*

Review, 6(1), 11–24. https://doi.org/10.1016/j.jalz.2009.10.002

Salthouse, T. A., Mitchell, D. R. D., Skovronek, E., & Babcock, R. L. (1989). Effects of adult
age and working memory on reasoning and spatial abilities. *Journal of Experimental
Psychology: Learning, Memory, and Cognition, 15*(3), 507–516.
https://doi.org/10.1037/0278-7393.15.3.507

Shaw, S., & Hoeber, L. (2003). "A strong man is direct and a direct woman is a bitch": Gendered
discourses and their influence on employment roles in sports organizations. *Journal of Sport
Management, 17*(4), 347–376.

Smart, C. M., Karr, J. E., Areshenkoff, C. N., Rabin, L. A., Hudon, C., Gates, N., … Wesselman,
L. (2017). Non-Pharmacologic interventions for older adults with subjective cognitive
decline: Systematic review, meta-analysis, and preliminary recommendations.
Neuropsychology Review, 27(3), 245–257. https://doi.org/10.1007/s11065-017-9342-8

Smart, C. M., & Krawitz, A. (2015). The impact of subjective cognitive decline on Iowa
Gambling Task performance. *Neuropsychology, 29*(6), 971–987.
https://doi.org/10.1037/neu0000204

Stewart, R., Russ, C., Richards, M., Brayne, C., Lovestone, S., & Mann, A. (2001). Depression,
APOE genotype and subjective memory impairment: A cross-sectional study in an African-
Caribbean population. *Psychological Medicine, 31*(3), 431–440.

Weintraub, S., Besser, L., Dodge, H. H., Teylan, M., Ferris, S., Goldstein, F. C., … Morris, J. C.
(2018). Version 3 of the Alzheimer Disease Centers' neuropsychological test battery in the
Uniform Data Set (UDS). *Alzheimer Disease and Associated Disorders, 32*(1), 10–17.
https://doi.org/10.1097/WAD.0000000000000223

Tables

Table 4.1. Neuropsychological assessment battery and self-report measures

Administered Tests/Measures

Neuropsychological Assessment Battery
    Animal Naming Test
    Boston Naming Test, 2nd edition
    California Verbal Learning Test, 2nd edition
    Controlled Oral Word Association Test
    Golden Stroop Test
    Test of Practical Judgment
    Trailmaking Test A and B
    Wechsler Advanced Clinical Solutions for the WAIS-IV and WMS-IV: Test of Premorbid Function
    Wechsler Adult Intelligence Scale, 4th edition: Digit Span
    Wechsler Memory Scale, 4th edition: Logical Memory I and II
    Wechsler Memory Scale, 4th edition: Visual Reproduction I and II

Self-report Measures
    Adult Manifest Anxiety Scale, elderly version (AMAS-E)
    Geriatric Depression Scale (GDS)
    UCLA Loneliness Scale

Table 4.2. Participant demographics

	Healthy Control n=40		Subtle Cognitive Decline n=25	
	No Concern n=27	SCD n=13	No Concern n=16	SCD n=9
General				
Female n (%)	21 (77.78)	11 (84.62)	12 (75.00)	7 (77.78)
Age M (SD)	74.96 (6.41)	75.46 (7.63)	70.19 (4.45)	75.22 (4.12)
Yrs Education M (SD)	16.15 (2.71)	16.31 (2.29)	15.00 (3.16)	15.78 (3.23)
Family dementia Hx n (%)	10 (37.04)	9 (69.23)	5 (31.25)	2 (22.22)
Mental Health Hx				
Depression n (%)	7 (25.93)	5 (38.46)	4 (25.00)	2 (22.22)
Anxiety n (%)	3 (11.11)	1 (7.69)	1 (6.25)	2 (22.22)
PTSD n (%)	1 (3.70)	1 (7.69)	0 (0.00)	0 (0.00)
Physical Health Hx				
Cancer n (%)	5 (18.52)	5 (38.46)	4 (25.00)	3 (33.33)
Diabetes n (%)	4 (14.82)	1 (7.69)	1 (6.25)	1 (11.11)
Heart problems n (%)	7 (25.93)	3 (23.08)	2 (12.50)	0 (0.00)
High blood pressure n (%)	7 (25.93)	4 (30.77)	2 (12.50)	1 (11.11)
High cholesterol n (%)	9 (33.33)	0 (0.00)	2 (12.50)	1 (11.11)

Table 4.3. Code descriptions and exemplar quotes

Coded Content	Code Description	Exemplar Quote
General Memory Strategies	Non-descript implementation of memory strategies.	"I rely on strategies a little bit more. Because it's hard to keep it all in your mind but with those strategies you're pretty okay."
Notes, Records, Calendars	Documenting information for later review.	"Yeah, sometimes I write stuff down. Sometimes, you know, I would make a mental note of it but I would, at this point prefer to write it down now because my time is limited."
Avoiding Multitasking	Deliberate or spontaneous reduction of divided attention/switching demands.	"I mean I have to do one thing at a time, and when, when I, when I start getting into some mulitasking mode, it just- like everything just falls apart. Everything just falls apart, so now I really try to concentrate, not to do multitasking."
Organizational Strategies	Deliberate efforts to order one's surroundings to reduce stress.	"You know it's kind of like, uhm, I don't know and I'm finding I ...I need more order than I did in the past."
Preparing for Decline	Preparing advanced medical directives etc. and generally making efforts to ensure a smooth transition into later life.	"So I did make up papers, of, a representative agreement for my daughter, so that she can put me away even if I'm kicking and screaming. And power of attorney, and I've done all those things, just in case those things happen."
Researching Aging	Reading books and academic articles related to dementia and age-related cognitive/ and/or physical decline.	"I have a suspicion that it must have from what I've read about the differences in, there's a lot of other people looking at this and I've read articles about it and they've identified certain kinds of cognitive abilities that seem to get better and others that get worse, those are the articles that I've read."
Repetition and Rehearsal	Mentally repeating information to ensure its maintenance in working memory.	"You have a phone number or somebody gives you a phone number and you have to enter it into the thing, I'm telling myself the phone number as I walk to the phone repeating it in my head, not just trusting that I'll remember it's 250 whatever whatever, you know.
Rereading/Reviewing Material	Repeatedly revisiting written information to ensure its maintenance in memory.	"Sometimes I have to read things twice."
Skimming for Gist	Perfunctorily scanning written information for standout phrases or points at the expense of careful study.	"I think I don't take in stuff as readily as... when I'm reading as readily as I used to .. I tend to sort of skim over it and then realize, 'wait a minute you read all that but you didn't take it in.'"

Coded Content	Code Description	Exemplar Quote
Absent-mindedness	Inattention or "mind-blanking".	"I feel sometimes, 'huh, what I've done?' Forty-five minutes have gone by and I'm still half looking for that thing and actually thinking about people I should contact, and not really being so focused on the one thing that I really would like to maybe see accomplished."
Effortful attention	Increased effort required to focus or maintain attention.	"I really need to keep my mind on the driving and not let my brain go off in to a hundred different directions... which it is a change... I really have to focus on it."
Distractibility	Having attention easily disrupted by external stimuli.	"I guess I can be distracted more readily than when I was young. Uh so if I'm got a task to do and something is impacted I might turn away from the task in order to pay attention to that, whereas I'd be more focused as a young man."
Divided attention	Attending to/monitoring multiple tasks simultaneously, multi-tasking.	"Well I noticed that umm I don't multitask as well, I don't remember umm you know a half a dozen things all at the same time."
Cognitive fatigue	Exhaustion or a sense of energy depletion following cognitive demand.	"I used to be able to sit down and get my lectures ready and i would thoroughly prepare my lectures and I used to be able to do that in a shorter amount of time and now I feel that I sometimes need to recoup."
Keeping up with Conversation	Ability to remain fully engaged in fluid conversations and rapid social exchanges.	"Sorry, sometimes it's really frustrating because sometimes you pause and you don't really get to finish the conversation because, you've blown it. It doesn't come to me so they say, 'well we have to move on, talk about something else.'"
Losing track of activity	Forgetting what one set out to do.	"I go into a room and I wonder what I went in for. I've forgotten!"
Misplacing items	Misplacing items or losing track of where objects were placed.	"I occasionally forget where I've parked the car, which never happened before, and I have to kind of think back... and that's a new thing."
Losing track of story plot	Losing the thread of a narrative, perhaps leading one to review material before continuing.	"I've got to remind myself. Ah, so I have to go back and think, 'oh yes, oh yeah that happened" and then I don't really go the whole chapter I get the "oh yeah that happened" and...then I...then I go on. Yeah, it gives me enough information...that I can go on.
Losing track of topic	Difficulty monitoring topic of conversation as the focus shifts/develops.	"Sometimes things just go missing. Like we think... I can't remember... like right now I can't remember exactly what we were talking about."

Coded Content	Code Description	Exemplar Quote
Memory for appointments	Ability to recall appointments or dates.	"I missed a couple of appointments or double scheduled a few things. And I'm sure it happened in the past too, not that often… Now it seems to happen more often."
Memory for conversations	Ability to recall conversations.	"My wife will say from time to time, 'well I told you this a couple of days ago.' I have no recollection whatever of that being told to me. So I have to believe that she actually did or somehow it didn't strike me or something."
Learning new information	Ability to encode information efficiently and reliably.	"It requires considerably more time to learn something, and it may require this sort of older method of going through it three or four times."
Episodic memory (proximal)	Ability to recall recent lived events.	"Recent memory is nowhere near as good as, uh, ancient memory."
Episodic memory (remote)	Ability to recall distant lived events.	"People have talked about an incident that I was involved in and I have no memory of it. And uh, that's happened maybe more frequently."
General memory	Non-descript statements regarding memory as a whole.	"I think my memory is going a bit."
Memory for names	Recalling names previously known.	"I know the people, I remember events, I can remember things in my own life but the names often escape me."
Semantic memory	Recalling information previously known.	"Probably some [memories] are disappearing. We watch Jeopardy from time to time and uh… pretty good. Maybe not quite as good as I would've… I was."
Rumination/mind wandering	Perseveration, or attentional interference due to preoccupation with unrelated events or issues.	"It's like something beams in that says, 'oh!' You know, thoughts that are not related to what I should be focused on come drifting in."
Processing speed	The speed and efficiency of processing incoming information.	"I don't think I'm quite as quick."

Coded Content	Code Description	Exemplar Quote
Word-finding	Recalling/delivering words in the moment.	"Well certainly when you're searching for that word or the name of that person, I think, 'damn it's taking a while,' and we're in the middle of the conversation and I want to mention the name, refer to them, and that word just doesn't come 'til much later."
Orientation/ navigation	Navigating to, from, and within familiar environments.	"One day I took a wrong turn in my car, and I did get back to where I wanted to – where I was going – but I sort of panicked because, I'd taken the wrong turn and that led me to this place and this place… places I hadn't ever been to or hadn't seen for a long time. I did eventually make it but I would've been better earlier on."
Activity derailment	Having one's intended action subverted by exposure to novel stimuli, especially those cueing a competing task.	"Something else like I'm working on something, have to answer the phone, that's happening, then I realize I have to go to the bathroom and a whole bunch of stuff and it's just like [sighs] then I start to get into that panic mode. Then everything starts to like, 'my God, please!'"
Reorienting after interruption	Resuming one's task following a disruption or brief interval.	"Then the phone rings or something happens and stuff like that and I go and take care of that then it's hard to get back into that [original task]."
Working memory	Maintaining information in mind for the time required to act on it.	"Uhm yeah I'd say definitely not as good. It's just like I can.. if I do go out without that shopping list it can be a challenge and I'd forget at least one of the things. Another thing that might be comparable in a way is uhm I know most people don't use telephone books anymore, but I still do. You know, if I'm looking up – I used to have absolutely no trouble at all keeping the number in mind and going off and dialing it whereas now, if it's more than a few seconds between doing those few things, then I'd have trouble with it."
Sequencing	Completing tasks in an organized and efficient chronological order.	"I put it [the milk] away and then I had to get it out again because I hadn't done both jobs with the milk at one time. I did one, put it away, looked for the milk, 'oh Hell, it's not there.'"
Sustained attention	Maintaining focus on a task or stimulus for a prolonged period of time.	"I think I have lost the ability to concentrate for long periods. I used to be able to study a problem for hours and hours and solve it. Now I need more instant gratification, I think."
Switching	Shifting attention from stimulus to stimulus deliberately and as required.	"But I noticed that I wasn't able to, uh, do as many tasks as I used to be able to do. Um, and then I remember them, and then I go back and do them. And I guess I do that now. But, you know, like, leave the bathwater running and then get absorbed in something else and then go, 'oh my God!' You know? 'I left the water running in the bathtub!' Okay, so those things I have noticed over the past five or six years."

Coded Content	Code Description	Exemplar Quote
Tangentiality/ circumstantiality	Speaking in an overly-inclusive, roundabout manner and/or demonstrating difficulty remaining on the relevant topic of discussion.	"I think sometimes I know what I want to talk about, and you get a little sidetracked. And then I usually notice that and I try to come back to what I'm saying. So its a little detour, sometimes, and I'm actually quite glad if people say 'hey, we were talking about this and not that.'"

Table 4.4. Codes per category and theme

Theme 1: Cognitive Change

	Attention/ Processing Decline	Executive Function Decline	Memory Decline	Language Decline	Visuospatial Processing Decline	**Total Decline**
Coded Content						
Absent-mindedness*	X					X
Effortful attention*	X					X
Distractibility*	X					X
Divided attention		X				X
Cognitive fatigue*	X					X
Keeping up with conversation	X	X		X		X
Losing track of activity*	X	X				X
Misplacing items*	X					X
Losing track of story plot*		X				X
Losing track of topic*	X			X		X
Memory for appointments		X	X			X
Memory for conversations			X			X
Learning new information			X			X
Episodic memory (proximal)			X			X
Episodic memory (remote)			X			X
General memory			X			X
Memory for names			X	X		X
Semantic memory			X			X
Word-finding			X	X		X
Orientation/navigation					X	X
Rumination/mind wandering*	X					X
Processing speed	X					X
Activity derailment*		X				X
Reorienting after interruption		X				X
Working memory		X				X
Sequencing		X				X
Sustained attention	X					X
Switching		X				X
Tangentiality/circumstantiality*		X		X		X

Theme 2: Behavioural Change

	Anticipating Decline	Reducing Cognitive Load	Organizing Environment	Increasing Exposure	Total Strategies
Coded Content					
General Memory Strategies*			X		X
Notes, Records, Calendars*			X		X
Avoiding Multitasking*		X			X
Organizational Strategies*			X		X
Preparing for Decline*	X				X
Researching Aging*	X				X
Repetition and Rehearsal*				X	X
Rereading/Reviewing Material*				X	X
Skimming for Gist*		X			X

* reported increase in frequency or intensity

Table 4.5. Code and category endorsement description

	Healthy Control n=40		Subtle Cognitive Decline n=25	
	No Concern n=27	SCD n=13	No Concern n=16	SCD n=9
Theme 1: Cognitive Change				
Coded Content				
Absent-mindedness n (%)	1 (3.70)	1 (7.69)	2 (12.50)	1 (11.11)
Effortful attention n (%)	4 (14.82)	7 (53.85)	4 (25.00)	0 (0.00)
Distractibility n (%)	2 (7.41)	2 (15.39)	5 (31.25)	3 (33.33)
Divided attention n (%)	8 (29.63)	6 (46.15)	3 (18.75)	3 (33.33)
Cognitive fatigue n (%)	3 (11.11)	3 (23.08)	3 (18.75)	2 (22.22)
Keeping up with conversation n (%)	2 (7.41)	3 (23.08)	0 (0.00)	1 (11.11)
Losing track of activity n (%)	13 (48.15)	9 (69.23)	4 (25.00)	5 (55.56)
Misplacing items n (%)	6 (22.22)	3 (23.08)	4 (25.00)	0 (0.00)
Losing track of story plot n (%)	1 (3.70)	3 (23.08)	1 (6.25)	0 (0.00)
Losing track of topic n (%)	3 (11.11)	0 (0.00)	0 (0.00)	2 (22.22)
Memory for appointments n (%)	5 (18.52)	3 (23.08)	1 (6.25)	2 (22.22)
Memory for conversations n (%)	2 (7.41)	0 (0.00)	0 (0.00)	3 (33.33)
Learning new information n (%)	10 (37.03)	6 (46.15)	6 (37.50)	5 (55.56)
Episodic memory (proximal) n (%)	2 (7.41)	3 (23.08)	4 (25.00)	2 (22.22)
Episodic memory (remote) n (%)	4 (14.82)	4 (30.77)	1 (6.25)	1 (11.11)
General memory n (%)	4 (14.82)	2 (15.39)	1 (6.25)	1 (11.11)
Memory for names n (%)	4 (14.82)	3 (23.08)	2 (12.50)	3 (33.33)
Semantic memory n (%)	5 (18.52)	4 (30.77)	1 (6.25)	1 (11.11)
Word-finding n (%)	20 (74.07)	8 (61.54)	12 (75.00)	8 (88.89)
Orientation/navigation n (%)	4 (14.82)	2 (15.39)	0 (0.00)	2 (22.22)
Rumination/mind wandering n (%)	6 (22.22)	3 (23.08)	2 (12.50)	3 (33.33)
Processing speed n (%)	12 (44.44)	5 (38.46)	6 (37.50)	3 (33.33)
Activity derailment n (%)	7 (25.93)	6 (46.15)	2 (12.50)	1 (11.11)
Reorienting after interruption n (%)	4 (14.82)	3 (23.08)	1 (6.25)	2 (22.22)
Working memory n (%)	10 (37.03)	10 (76.92)	4 (25.00)	5 (55.56)
Sequencing n (%)	3 (11.11)	0 (0.00)	0 (0.00)	3 (33.33)
Sustained attention n (%)	6 (22.22)	1 (7.69)	4 (25.00)	1 (11.11)
Switching n (%)	8 (29.63)	9 (69.23)	8 (50.00)	4 (44.44)
Tangentiality/circumstantiality n (%)	0 (0.00)	3 (23.08)	3 (18.75)	1 (11.11)

	Healthy Control n=40		Subtle Cognitive Decline n=25	
	No Concern n=27	SCD n=13	No Concern n=16	SCD n=9
Theme 1: Cognitive Change				
Combined Categories				
Attention/Processing Decline M (SD)	2.15 (1.46)	2.85 (1.46)	2.13 (1.89)	2.33 (1.23)
Executive Function Decline M (SD)	2.26 (1.48)	4.23 (1.48)	1.69 (1.14)	3.00 (1.12)
Memory Decline M (SD)	2.07 (1.27)	2.54 (1.05)	1.75 (1.29)	2.89 (1.76)
Language Decline M (SD)	1.07 (0.73)	1.31 (1.11)	1.06 (0.68)	1.67 (0.71)
Visuospatial Processing Decline M (SD)	0.15 (0.36)	0.15 (0.38)	0 (0.00)	0.22 (0.44)
Total Cognitive Decline M (SD)	5.89 (2.76)	8.62 (2.47)	5.25 (2.62)	7.56 (2.70)
Theme 2: Behavioural Change				
Coded Content				
General Memory Strategies n (%)	2 (7.41)	2 (15.38)	2 (12.50)	1 (11.11)
Notes, Records, Calendars n (%)	10 (37.04)	10 (76.92)	6 (37.50)	5 (55.56)
Avoiding Multitasking n (%)	8 (29.63)	8 (61.54)	3 (18.75)	4 (44.44)
Organizational Strategies n (%)	3 (11.11)	1 (7.69)	2 (12.50)	2 (22.22)
Preparing for Decline n (%)	2 (7.41)	0 (0.00)	1 (6.25)	2 (22.22)
Researching Aging n (%)	0 (0.00)	3 (23.08)	1 (6.25)	2 (22.22)
Repetition and Rehearsal n (%)	2 (7.41)	5 (38.46)	0 (0.00)	1 (11.11)
Rereading/Reviewing Material n (%)	3 (11.11)	2 (15.38)	1 (6.25)	3 (33.33)
Skimming for Gist n (%)	2 (7.41)	2 (15.38)	3 (18.75)	1 (11.11)
Combined Categories				
Anticipating Decline M (SD)	0.07 (0.27)	0.23 (0.44)	0.13 (0.34)	0.44 (0.73)
Reducing Cognitive Load M (SD)	0.37 (0.49)	0.77 (0.60)	0.38 (0.50)	0.56 (0.73)
Organizing Environment M (SD)	0.56 (0.70)	1.00 (0.58)	0.63 (0.50)	0.89 (0.60)
Increasing Exposure M (SD)	0.19 (0.40)	0.54 (0.52)	0.06 (0.25)	0.44 (0.73)
Total Compensatory Strategies M (SD)	1.19 (0.88)	2.54 (1.05)	1.19 (0.91)	2.33 (1.66)

Table 4.6. MANOVA effects on total codes endorsed per category

	SCD			Subtle Cognitive Decline			SCD X Subtle Cognitive Decline		
	F-value	p-value	ηp^2	F-value	p-value	ηp^2	F-value	p-value	ηp^2
Omnibus: Wilks' λ	1.285	.284	.149	1.473	.210	.167	.327	.919	.043
Theme 1: Cognitive Change									
Attention/Processing Decline	.899	.348	.018	.494	.486	.010	.427	.516	.009
Executive Function Decline	**7.183**	**.010**	**.128**	**5.520**	**.023**	**.101**	.555	.460	.011
Memory Decline	.588	.447	.012	.004	.947	.000	.294	.590	.006
Language Decline*	-	.103	-	-	.526	-	.800	.375	.016
Visuospatial Processing Decline*	-	.306	-	-	.407	-	1.602	.212	.032
Total Cognitive Decline	**4.446**	**.040**	**.083**	1.126	.294	.022	.103	.749	.002
Theme 2: Behavioural Change									
Anticipating Decline*	-	.054	-	-	.389	-	-	-	-
Reducing Cognitive Load	1.055	.309	.021	0.233	.632	.005	0.707	.405	.014
Organizing Environment	1.111	.297	.022	0.288	.594	.006	0.024	.879	.000
Increasing Exposure*	-	**.005**	-	-	.249	-	-	-	-
Total Compensatory Strategies*	-	**.000**	-	-	.680	-	-	-	-

*Analyzed via Mann-Whitney U test; **Bold**: significant at $p<.05$; *Italic*: found not to be significant following post-hoc analysis.

Appendix

Table 4.A1. Covariate *p*-values on total codes endorsed per category

	Age	Sex	Yrs Ed.	Familial Dementia	Psych Dx	GDS	LON	AMAS WOS	AMAS PHYS	AMAS FEAR	AMAS LIE	AMAS Total
Omnibus: Wilks' λ	.820	.698	.077	.920	.820	.833	.340	.282	.481	.915	.817	.463
Theme 1: Cognitive Change												
Attention/Processing Decline	.316	.524	.203	.735	.871	.318	.678	.839	.902	.738	.126	.820
Executive Function Decline	.914	.475	.706	.505	.713	.897	.314	.396	.793	.489	.461	.278
Memory Decline	.525	.600	.800	.833	.301	.874	.712	.151	.953	.664	.582	.279
Language Decline*	-	-	-	-	-	-	-	-	-	-	-	-
Visuospatial Processing Decline*	-	-	-	-	-	-	-	-	-	-	-	-
Total Cognitive Decline	.845	.967	.497	.797	.601	.604	.991	.290	.567	.379	.408	.206
Theme 2: Behavioural Change												
Anticipating Decline*	-	-	-	-	-	-	-	-	-	-	-	-
Reducing Cognitive Load	.445	.695	.996	.793	.251	.995	.653	.521	.629	.775	.988	.556
Organizing Environment	.845	.365	**.010**	.963	.458	.438	.067	**.017**	.124	.746	.959	.051
Increasing Exposure*	-	-	-	-	-	-	-	-	-	-	-	-
Total Compensatory Strategies*	-	-	-	-	-	-	-	-	-	-	-	-

*Covariate data unavailable due to substitution of MANOVA with Mann-Whitney *U* test; **Bold**: significant at *p*<.05

Multimodal risk profiles for pathological cognitive decline

Table 4.A2. Semi-structured interview schedule

Key Item	Possible Queries (phrasing may vary)
Tell me about your **thinking abilities** as you have gotten older?	(Q) In the past 5 years or so? (Q) What, if anything, has gotten more challenging for you? (Q) What, if anything, has gotten easier for you? (Q) What, if anything, has stayed the same for you?
How has your **processing speed** been (e.g., the speed with which you are able to think and process information)? *Provide examples as necessary*	(Q) What has changed (as you have gotten older/in the past 5 years)? (Q) What is just as it has always been? (Q) How about your ability to keep up with conversations? (Q) How about your ability to notice and respond to things? (Q) Has that gotten in the way of your doing the things you would like to/are used to doing? …How has that gotten in the way/what has that gotten in the way of? (Q) What do you do to help yourself keep up (better)?
How has your **attention** been? *Provide examples as necessary*	(Q) What has changed (as you have gotten older/in the past 5 years)? (Q) What is just as it has always been? (Q) How about your ability to focus on things? (Q) How about your ability to concentrate for longer periods of time? (Q) Do you feel you are more distractible? …By external stimuli (e.g., sounds, etc.)? …By internal stimuli (e.g., preoccupied by worries, etc.)? (Q) Do you find paying attention takes more effort than before? (Q) Has that gotten in the way of your doing the things you would like to/are used to doing? …How has that gotten in the way/what has that gotten in the way of? (Q) What do you do to help yourself pay attention more (easily)?

Multimodal risk profiles for pathological cognitive decline

Key Item	Possible Queries (phrasing may vary)
How has your **working memory** been (e.g., your ability to keep information in mind for a time)? *Provide examples as necessary*	(Q) What has changed (as you have gotten older/in the past 5 years)? (Q) What is just as it has always been? (Q) How about your ability to keep information in mind for a short time? (Q) How about your ability to keep track of what you were doing? (Q) Has that gotten in the way of your doing the things you would like to/are used to doing? …How has that gotten in the way/what has that gotten in the way of? (Q) What do you do to help yourself keep information in mind (better)?
How has your **memory** been (e.g., learning and recall)? *Provide examples as necessary*	(Q) What has changed (as you have gotten older/in the past 5 years)? (Q) What is just as it has always been? (Q) How about your ability to learn new information? (Q) Do you find learning takes more effort than before? (Q) How about your ability remember things? …Events from the distant past? …Events from the recent past? …Information that you know/once knew well? …Names? …Activities? (Q) How about your ability to remember dates and appointments? (Q) How about your ability to remember to do things later? (Q) Has that gotten in the way of your doing the things you would like to/are used to doing? …How has that gotten in the way/what has that gotten in the way of? (Q) What do you do to help yourself learn/remember more (easily)?

Multimodal risk profiles for pathological cognitive decline

Key Item	Possible Queries (phrasing may vary)
How has your **language** been (e.g., your ability to understand and communicate)? *Provide examples as necessary*	(Q) What has changed (as you have gotten older/in the past 5 years)? (Q) What is just as it has always been? (Q) How about your ability to understand when people are speaking to you? …How about if your hearing was 100%. How would it be, then? (Q) How about your ability to communicate clearly? …Has there been any change in your ability to stay on topic? …Has there been any change in how direct you are in your speech? (Q) How about your ability to find the right word at the right time? (Q) Has that gotten in the way of your doing the things you would like to/are used to doing? …How has that gotten in the way/what has that gotten in the way of? (Q) What do you do to help yourself understand/communicate (more clearly)?
How has your **visuospatial functioning** been (e.g., navigation/orientation)? *Provide examples as necessary*	(Q) What has changed (as you have gotten older/in the past 5 years)? (Q) What is just as it has always been? (Q) How about your ability to find your way to/in familiar locations? (Q) How about your ability to find your way back when you get turned around/lost? (Q) Has that gotten in the way of your doing the things you would like to/are used to doing? …How has that gotten in the way/what has that gotten in the way of? (Q) What do you do to help yourself navigate?

Multimodal risk profiles for pathological cognitive decline

Key Item	Possible Queries (phrasing may vary)
How has your **executive functioning** been (e.g., multitasking, problem-solving)? *Provide examples as necessary*	(Q) What has changed (as you have gotten older/in the past 5 years)? (Q) What is just as it has always been? (Q) How about your ability to multitask? …How about doing several things at the same time? …How about switching back and forth between tasks? (Q) How about your ability to problem-solve? (Q) How about your ability to make (good) decisions? (Q) Have you become more impulsive over time? (Q) Have you noticed difficulties "switching gears"? (Q) Have you noticed difficulties with planning or carrying out activities in a specific sequence? (Q) Has that gotten in the way of your doing the things you would like to/are used to doing? …How has that gotten in the way/what has that gotten in the way of? (Q) What do you do to help yourself multitask/stay on top of things (better)?
How has your **mood** been? *Provide examples as necessary*	(Q) What has changed (as you have gotten older/in the past 5 years)? (Q) What is just as it has always been? (Q) Has your mood declined more/been lower? (Q) Have you felt more anxious? …Do you find it difficult to turn off your worries? …Do you feel overwhelmed? (Q) Has that gotten in the way of your doing the things you would like to/are used to doing? …How has that gotten in the way/what has that gotten in the way of? (Q) What do you do to help yourself navigate?

Multimodal risk profiles for pathological cognitive decline

Key Item	Possible Queries (phrasing may vary)
How often does that happen for you? (for all reported areas of change)	(Q) Is that a change from before? (Q) How do you feel about that?
Does that cause you any **concern**? (for all reported areas of change) *Differentiate concern from change or functional disruption as necessary*	(Q) How do you feel about that? (Q) Do those changes make you worried? …What are you worried about? (Q) Do you think these changes are pathological? …What do you think might be happening? …Do you think these are expected changes for older adults?

247

General Discussion: Qualitatively-Informed Contributions to Early Dementia Risk Assessment

General Discussion

Neuropsychological assessment is a mixed-methods endeavor by its very nature. While standardized cognitive-neuropsychological tests and nomothetic comparisons may supply the most rigorous data, clinical interpretation of said outcomes cannot be divorced from the grander context of individuals' lived experiences. Indeed, the entire *meaning* of a given score may change depending on individual's circumstances, expectations, history, and other factors. For this reason, patient interviews are viewed as an absolutely integral part of ethical neuropsychological assessment. Unfortunately, (neuropsychological) research has not always remained consistent with these tenets of clinical practice. Research investigations often pertain to medical conditions and, consequently, may be seated within a greater medical context. As a result, our research into mild cognitive impairment (MCI), Alzheimer's disease (AD), and other objective cognitive impairment often reflects a concrete and quantitatively-driven approach. While there are clear merits to developing replicable and reliable cut-off scores and practice guidelines, an important, and arguably central, source of information is frequently disregarded: the patient's own experience of their condition and themselves. Thus, bearing this in mind, and as a book in clinical neuropsychology, the current work serves as an early step in bridging the qualitative-quantitative divide and aims to extend the principles of holistic neuropsychological assessment practice to the research domain. Further, a guiding objective of this work was to establish patients' voices as viable and worthwhile sources of clinical information.

With respect to these overarching objectives, we conducted a mixed-methods investigation of several well-established potential risk factors for objective pathological cognitive decline in later age. Chapter 1 presented a previously-published systematic review of the current evidence regarding the role of APOE ε4 genotype and subjective cognitive decline (SCD; Ali, Smart, &

Gawryluk, 2018). Chapter 2 presented the research methods and materials used for this book study. Chapter 3 introduced the first study conducted for the purposes of this book. In that investigation, we aimed to determine which demographic, psychosocial, and other factors relate most to the endorsement of SCD and the demonstration of objective, yet sub-clinical, subtle cognitive decline (subtle CD) on standardized cognitive-neuropsychological testing. As part of this goal, we aimed to determine whether SCD and subtle CD related to one another. Despite our *a priori* intention to test our Chapter 1 (i.e., systematic review) findings and examine the genetic contribution to SCD and subtle CD, APOE ε4 genotype was excluded from our analyses due to low representation of APOE ε4-positive genotype in our sample. Chapter 3 introduced a qualitative component to our work by investigating the relationship of SCD and subtle CD to self-reported experiences of cognitive change and behavioural compensation. More specifically, we collected qualitative interview data in the style of standard neuropsychological assessment with the goal of parsing which disclosures may be most suggestive of potential underlying cognitive risk.

Summary of Findings

In Chapter 3, SCD and subtle CD demonstrated unique relationships with various demographic factors and indicators of self-reported cognitive change. SCD endorsement was best predicted by increased anxiety regarding aging and age-related changes, self-perceived word-finding declines, and more general self-perceived cognitive declines. In contrast, subtle CD related most to self-reported declines in planning ability, greater anxiety regarding health and physiological functioning, and *lower* depressive symptomology – though this last was considered likely to result from statistical artifact.

Chapter 4 presented the effects of SCD and subtle CD on the endorsement of specific (categories of) qualitative experiences. Qualitative experiences were divided across two larger themes: cognitive change and behavioural change. With regard to cognitive changes, those reporting SCD endorsed significantly more executive functioning deficits than unconcerned older adults. On the other hand, those with subtle CD endorsed significantly *fewer* executive functioning deficits versus healthy controls. As may be expected, SCD endorsers reported significantly more cognitive declines than those who were unconcerned. Less expected was the null effect of subtle CD on the endorsement of cognitive declines. Expanding this further, those with SCD endorsed behavioural changes (e.g., engaging in compensatory strategies) significantly more than unconcerned older adults. The behavioural changes endorsed tended to be specific to strategies for maintaining information in working memory, such as rehearsal, review, and repetition.

Clinical Implications

The combined results of these studies present several important considerations for clinical practice and research. Synthesis of our various outcomes and interpretations provides several key points: 1) SCD and subtle CD reflect distinct constructs and unique sources of information that may relate to cognitive vulnerability; 2) the relationship between self-reported function and objective cognitive performance may vary according to degree of cognitive decline, degree of functional disruption and/or visibility of decline, or other psychosocial factors; and 3) with regard to early screening, executive functioning may represent a central cognitive domain of interest among those with risk factors for pathological cognitive decline.

SCD and subtle CD as distinct contributors to potential risk. Importantly, our Chapter 3 results suggest that SCD and subtle CD may contribute separable variance to the overall picture of cognitive change and functioning in healthy older adults. SCD and subtle CD were not identified as significant predictors of each other and, perhaps more importantly, did not directly share any predictor variables in common. At a high level, these outcomes resonate with previous findings that SCD reliably and primarily reflects personality and psychosocial factors rather than objective cognitive performance (Comijs, Deeg, Dik, Twisk, & Jonker, 2002; Derouesné, Lacomblez, Thibault, & LePoncin, 1999; Dux et al., 2008; Haavisto, 2018; Jenkins, Tree, Thornton, & Tales, 2019; Merema, Speelman, Foster, & Kaczmarek, 2013; Pearman & Storandt, 2005; Slavin et al., 2010; Snitz et al., 2015). However, it is important to note that, despite this, individuals endorsing SCD may still experience cognitive declines; however, any such declines may be too early in their progression and, consequently, too slight for standardized cognitive-neuropsychological tests to register. Indeed, experimental approaches have been successful in identifying cognitive decrements in those with SCD that were overlooked by standardized clinical tests (Mulligan, Smart, & Ali, 2016; Smart & Krawitz, 2015). Taken as a whole, this evidence suggests that, while it remains unclear whether, when, and to what extent older adults with SCD experience objective cognitive changes, it is clear that psychosocial factors play a heavy role in its expression.

Although it is key for clinicians to understanding the import of situational and psychosocial influences on patients' self-reported functioning, the psychosocial contributions to SCD may be even more crucial to impart to patients themselves. Ironically, given that prolonged emotional distress is known to accelerate the onset of objective cognitive decline (Richard et al., 2013), it is entirely possible that individuals who experience pronounced cognitive concerns may unwittingly increase their risk of developing the very outcomes they fear most. The current state of the evidence is not clear enough to determine when SCD may be a reflection of incipient cognitive decline; however, there is a strong possibility that SCD may serve a precipitant function for many, regardless of underlying vulnerability. Considering that the specific predictors for SCD endorsement related to relatively common age-related changes (e.g., word-finding challenges) in our sample, supportive psychoeducation and normalization around cognitive aging and functional compensation may prove beneficial (e.g., Memory and Aging Program: Wiegand, Troyer, Gojmerac, & Murphy, 2013). This may be even more strongly recommended where older adults are socially isolated or have few same-aged peers to contextualize their own aging experiences.

The lack of cohesion between SCD endorsement and subtle CD bears reemphasis, as this conflicts with the assumption of a linear pathological progression from SCD to more objective changes like subtle CD (Jessen et al., 2014). Our findings suggest that subtle CD may represent a unique construct with potential relevance to early dementia screening. In contrast to SCD, subtle CD was best predicted by potential uncommonly-reported changes in cognitive functioning (i.e., sequencing) and concerns regarding loss of functional ability (i.e., AMAS-E physiological anxiety). Indeed, those with subtle CD were only likely to endorse concern/SCD when reported executive functioning declines visibly impacted daily activity. Combined, these results support Hill and coworkers' contention that the core anxiety underlying cognitive concern may be the perceived degradation of their functional independence and agency (Hill et al., 2016). Thus, to the extent that those with subtle CD feel threatened by the possibility of institutionalization or other curtailing of freedoms, they may be less forthcoming during screening or may avoid clinical consultation altogether. Similar to those with SCD, it is likely that patients demonstrating subtle CD may benefit from supportive psychoeducation around age-normative changes in activity and cognition; however, they may be more challenging to identify and recruit.

The role of self-report and response bias in SCD and subtle CD. Dementia risk screening may be complicated further by the inconsistent relationship of cognitive self-report and objective functioning as cognitive decline becomes more apparent. Our findings suggest that a prominent ingredient in SCD endorsement may be anxiety and a desire to have their concerns validated. This not only corresponds to previous findings (Hill et al., 2016; Tobiansky, Livingston,

& Mann, 1995), but may explain the demonstrated tendency of those with SCD to over-report cognitive declines relative to informants (Mulligan, Smart, & Ali, 2016) and even those with MCI (Edmonds, Delano-Wood, Galasko, Salmon, & Bondi, 2014). Armed with such evidence, it would seem a simple matter to conclude that those with SCD are particularly unreliable sources of information regarding their own ability; however, biased responding may not be relegated to those experiencing subjective change alone.

Individuals demonstrating objectively lower cognitive performance (e.g., subtle CD, MCI) may also demonstrated a propensity toward biased responding, though in the opposite direction as those with SCD. While anosognosia (i.e., unawareness of one's deficits) may increase objective cognitive declines progress (Reisberg & Gauthier, 2008), it is unlikely that this would account for underreporting among those with subtle CD. Any objective cognitive decrements in this group would necessarily be so slight as to fall within the range of normal performance. Rather than being driven by a lack of awareness, potentially biased reporting among those with subtle CD may instead stem from *increased* awareness of cognitive changes currently underway. To the extent that individuals feel threatened by the possibility of dementia and related losses of independence, those with subtle CD may engage in defensive denial and may underreport cognitive challenges, concerns, and changes in order to stave against having their feared outcomes confirmed (Beard & Neary, 2013; Lingler et al., 2006).

These considerations are not purely speculative, as evidenced by our findings. Interestingly, although endorsement of executive functioning (planning) decline on the ECog measure was uniquely predictive of subtle CD status, those with subtle CD were significantly less likely than those with SCD to endorse executive function decrements during interview. This is even more discrepant given that the majority of low cognitive scores in the subtle CD sample related to executive functioning items/measures. Although one might expect an increase in compensatory strategy use among those with subtle CD, we did not find any increase in behavioural changes at all. It is true that our statistical power was low; however, the convergence of this evidence raises the possibility that some degree of response bias may have affected subtle CD participants' qualitative reports. Combined, these results suggest that individuals with SCD and those with subtle CD may be motivated by different factors. Where individuals with SCD may vie for acknowledgement and validation of their concerns, those with subtle CD may shy from disclosing changes openly to ward against any potential reinforcement of their concerns. For this reason, informant reports may become more important sources of information as individuals are suspected of developing greater objective cognitive declines and/or as the level of concrete threat to their independence is increased (Mulligan et al., 2016).

What a given individual may be able/willing to endorse may also differ according to the method of data collection and the presumed *meaning* of specific changes. As alluded to previously, our sample of individuals with subtle CD appeared to be more open to reporting executive functioning declines on a standardized self-report measures than during in-person interview. While interview allows for more reframing, probing, reassurance, and discussion, it may also prove too confrontational for some participants – this, particularly when discussion centres around topics that may be personally threatening for individuals. Similarly, changes in navigation/orientation were almost uniformly and vociferously denied during interview regardless of group membership, and this may well have been due to the perceived risk of endorsement. Several participants noted during interview that they were aware that endorsement of visuospatial processing declines was a common indicator of AD or other pathological cognitive decline. During our consent procedures, several participants also voiced concerns regarding our ethical obligation to report potential driving risk. These factors are likely to have primed participants to deny changes in orientation during interview. Unfortunately, it is not clear whether decrements in this domain may have been endorsed more readily on a questionnaire due to our exclusion of the relevant section of the ECog measure from our assessment battery.

As with any assessment, it can be difficult to distinguish reticence to disclose from absence of symptoms. This challenge may be mitigated somewhat by designing assessments to be straightforward, non-threatening, and multimodal. Where engaging in an interview may be particularly valuable for those with SCD who often feel unvalidated or misunderstood, it may lead individuals to disclose less when they fear evaluation may lead to an intractable diagnosis or loss of freedom. Consequently, rather than engaging in conversation about cognitive change immediately, it may be recommended to rely primarily on standardized measures for initial data collection regarding patients' self-reported cognitive functioning and then to use their endorsed experiences as a springboard for further discussion. Not only may patients feel more open to disclosing on paper, but concrete and functional questionnaire items may prove more accessible for older adults and more easily interpretable for clinicians alike (Tuokko & Smart, 2018). This approach may also allow for the administration of validity scales and/or measures with various degrees of face validity to determine the likelihood of deliberate response bias. Additional interview follow-up may provide an opportunity to identify areas of discrepancy and other contextual issues that may influence the conceptualization of patient issues and ideal intervention options.

Executive functioning as a central domain of interest. Departing from the majority of SCD and cognitive decline literature, our findings indicate that declines in executive functioning – and not episodic memory – may provide the earliest indication of burgeoning cognitive changes.

However, our findings do not stand alone. Similar conclusions have been reached by a number of qualitative (Amariglio, Townsend, Grodstein, Sperling, & Rentz, 2011; Miebach, Wolfsgruber, Frommann, Buckley, & Wagner, 2018) and quantitative enquiries (Mulligan et al., 2016; Smart & Krawitz, 2015). Considered through a neuroanatomical lens, the sensitivity of executive functioning to early-stage cognitive changes seems plain given its functional pervasiveness and diversity, reliance on coordinated neural networks (Elliott, 2003; Rabinovici, Stephens, & Possin, 2015), and fundamental involvement in other cognitive functions. Nevertheless, executive functioning poses its own challenges as a dementia risk screening domain of interest. Fluid reasoning and executive functioning decrements are normative in later life (McNab et al., 2015), which makes it difficult to determine exactly where the risk threshold should lie. This is especially challenging given that our populations of interest at this ambiguous stage of potential cognitive decline perform within the normal range on standardized testing. Additionally, given that executive functions subsume a number of distinct cognitive functions, and that not all decline predictably with age (e.g., judgment, problem solving), further study will be required before executive functioning can be enshrined as the undisputed dementia risk indicator.

With that said, our findings and others' may guide the initial steps of this exploration. Self-reported challenges keeping up with conversation, encoding and recalling the details of past conversations, and inefficient planning and sequencing of daily activities, may present risk for objective cognitive decline in advance of more developed episodic memory and visuospatial processing impairments. Observed tangentiality, circumlocution, and losing track of topic during conversation may also represent executive declines associated with the development of more pronounced impairment (disorganized speech: Miebach et al., 2018).

Caveats and Limitations

Sample size. Our findings warrant several qualifications. A chief limitation in our study was a low *n*, which impacted our statistical power and the representation of certain variables (e.g., APOE ε4 genotype). This, in turn, restricted the scope of our analysis more than would have been hoped. Although our findings are broadly consistent with the current literature, our outcomes remain suggestive at best due to their inherent statistical volatility.

Sample characteristics. Aside from the size of our sample, however, our participants also represented a very specific population which may limit the generalizability of our results. The majority of our sample comprised former academics and professionals of Northern European ancestry who were in excellent physical health. Not only were our participants likely to enjoy a relatively high cognitive reserve and degree of privilege, but many chose to participate expressly because they were aware that they were aging in an exemplary manner relative to their peers. Paired with reports that peers with more cognitive challenge were reticent to participate, this suggests that our sample was singularly confident and healthy. Importantly, this manifested as a systematically atypical interpretation of "cognitive concern". Where "cognitive concern" in clinical samples is typically experienced as immediate and potentially pathological by older adults (Jessen et al., 2020), our SCD participants almost universally endorsed abstract, general and, in their opinion, normative concern that dementia may occur in the far future. This is likely to have increased the variability within our SCD group and simultaneously undermined the comparability of our participants' experiences with other (clinical) study samples.

Another notable feature of our predominantly professional/academic sample was that it was also primarily female (78.5%). It is unclear why this sampling bias may have occurred or how it may have impacted the results of our studies, though we may be able to extrapolate somewhat from the literature. It is possible that the small *n* of male participants in our study may reflect a gender-normative reticence to report "unfounded" concerns (Haussmann, Sauer, Birnbaum, & Donix, 2019). In turn, those men who did report SCD may have represented only a select and particularly concerned sub-sample from the greater community. Contrarily, our female participants may have been *less* prone to report cognitive concerns and mental health symptoms for various reasons. One powerful contextual factor may have been the larger sociohistorical factors and unique experiences of highly-educated professional women in this age cohort. Overcoming institutional obstacles to independence and success throughout their careers (e.g. cultures of sexism, reduced opportunities for advancement due to sex/gender, etc.) likely required women to develop a persona characterized by invulnerability and unquestionable competence (Friedman & Yorio, 2006; Shaw & Hoeber, 2003). As a result, it is possible that women in our sample may have been exceedingly reticent to disclose information that could possibly undermine their perceived agency, competence, or capacity to make decisions – this, especially when speaking with a younger male researcher.

As noted, it is difficult to determine what effect the uniqueness of our sample may have had on our outcomes. It is possible that the dynamic between older women and a younger male researcher may have impacted our data. Older women may have felt more comfortable disclosing areas of vulnerability, concern, or challenge with another woman of advanced age during interview. That said, speaking to a same-aged peer may also have raised the potential for interpersonal comparisons. It is difficult to know, however, it may be fair to assume that our participants may have been more guarded to the extent that they felt they would be misunderstood or reduced by disclosure, While female sex is a predominant characteristic of our sample, however, it is not the only trait that may have impacted our outcomes. For instance, our sample was highly educated and it has been shown that higher education increased the likelihood of SCD endorsement

(Tuokko & Smart, 2018). Those less identified with their cognitve functioning may well report fewer concerns. Those less-attuned to such changes may actually report few cognitive changes at all as their declines have not been disruptive to their usual activities. Similarly, those in more rural settings (compared to our urban sample) may value other areas of their functioning that relate more to familial/social roles or functional activities. Changes in higher-order areas like executive functioning may prove less bothersome for individuals who live according to simplified schedules and who value the quality of experience over productivity. Various other factors may likewise impart some degree of influence over our qualitative and self-report data. In order to understand and account for these influences, similar work with more diverse samples is crucial.

Variables of interest. Other caveats relate more to our constructs of interest and our determination of group membership. We made efforts to remain consistent with the SCD *Plus* guidelines established by the SCD-Initiative Working Group (Jessen et al., 2014) by querying cognitive concern and establishing the presence of self-reported cognitive change; nevertheless, we were unable to account for several other criteria that may have more soundly established a vulnerability to pathological cognitive decline. As mentioned previously, we were unable to meaningfully include APOE ε4 genotype in our calculations as there were few individuals with APOE ε4-positive genotype. We did collect informant reports when possible, however, there was considerable variability in informant availability, available informants' relationships to participants, and participants' willingness to include informants when they feared unfavourable reports. Due to the variability (noise) added by the inclusion of informant reports and the low *n* of informants overall, this source of information was also excluded.

Finally, subtle CD represented potential sub-clinical objective cognitive decrements in our studies. Although this construct has been supported as a risk factor for pathological cognitive decline in some respects (Edmonds, Delano-Wood, Galasko, Salmon, & Bondi, 2015; Sperling et al., 2011), its diagnostic sensitivity and specificity remain questionable. This is a particularly notable concern given that the current criteria for subtle CD (Edmonds et al., 2015) was generated theoretically rather than psychometrically. Although we revised these criteria for the purposes of the current study and for use with a comprehensive assessment battery, it remains unclear whether our general adherence to Edmonds et al.'s (2015) subtle CD criteria was too sensitive to normal test score variance or too insensitive to potential underlying neuropathology. Absent additional longitudinal studies of subtle CD, it is impossible to know whether our assumption of cognitive risk will be borne out over the longer term.

Recommendations for Future Research

Future extensions of this work would be well-served by several adjustments to study design and sampling to mitigate the limitations outlined above. As a cross-sectional study, the current work was limited in its ability to delineate participants' cognitive trajectories or substantiate the proposed vulnerability conferred by SCD and subtle CD. Longitudinal investigations that include a similar qualitative component at multiple time points may be ideal for determining the relationship of early risk factors and self-reported experiences on longer-term cognitive functioning. Further, longitudinal study may clarify how well subjective reports of functioning align with objective cognitive performance as time passes and cognitive ability changes. However, that is not to say that additional cross-sectional studies would be fruitless. Where longitudinal exploration is unfeasible, multiple cross-sectional studies representing a larger range of cognitive ability (e.g., SCD, subtle CD, MCI, AD) may approximate the developmental information provided by assessment at multiple time points. Another design consideration may be the counterbalancing of data collection activities to mitigate the potential impact of neuropsychological testing experiences on participants' cognitive self-evaluation during interview.

With regard to sampling, our study suffered from a relatively small and homogeneous participant pool, which impacted our statistical power and the generalizability of our results. The recruitment of a larger and more ethnically, socioeconomically, educationally, and sexually diverse sample would significantly strengthen this work. Although recruitment based purely on APOE ε4 genotype would be ill-advised, it is possible that a broad sample in other respects may reflect more relevant genetic variation as well. Additionally, direct comparison of clinical and community-based samples with SCD and/or subtle CD would also help to clarify which experiences may be more readily endorsed by older adults in various settings, with various degrees of cognitive concern, and with varying degrees of openness to medical intervention and/or corroboration.

The specific criteria used to determine SCD and subtle CD may also merit close attention as this work progresses. Our difficulties using a single item to determine SCD (i.e., atypical interpretation of "concern" within our sample) combined with evidence suggesting that SCD classification may differ according to criteria and method of determination (Vogel, Salem, Andersen, & Waldemar, 2016), indicate that the classification of SCD requires further attention and standardization. As a complement, it may be advantageous for future large-scale longitudinal studies to include multiple measures of SCD, as well as various sources of complementary risk-predicting data (e.g., genotype, informant reports). Doing so would not only provide valuable information regarding the convergent validity of various measures but may also clarify which conceptualization of SCD is most closely tied to specific cognitive outcomes. As a first step, a reliability analysis of various SCD classification methods may be warranted. Similarly, the construct of subtle CD may benefit from more refinement. It remains unclear whether our – or for that matter, Edmonds and coworkers' (Edmonds et al., 2015) – criteria is optimally sensitive to early cognitive perturbation. The continued use and psychometric value of subtle CD in early dementia risk research is recommended. As a start, larger studies may seek to determine an optimally predictive threshold of below-mean scores.

Finally, building upon our findings, future work seeking to identify ideal and early indicators of risk of pathological cognitive decline would do well to emphasize the assessment of subjective and objective executive functioning and language abilities to determine which specific functions (e.g., working memory, inhibition, switching) and what degree of change (e.g., diagnostic cut-off scores) are most clinically predictive.

Conclusion

The work presented in this book demonstrates that SCD and subtle CD may provide unique insights into current and potential cognitive functioning. It is possible that, where SCD most clearly reflects psychosocial vulnerabilities, subtle CD may instead reflect burgeoning functional disruptions. Our findings further indicate that executive function may be a key factor in early cognitive change. However, the data presented also raises important questions regarding the nature of patient disclosure, how to establish meaningful diagnostic thresholds, and how to reconcile differences between clinical and community-based samples of older adults for the purposes of continuing research. In pursuit of a better understanding of early-stage cognitive decline, we recommend that mixed-methods approaches be included as a matter of course in large-scale longitudinal studies. Further, we encourage replication and extension of this work with more cognitively, ethnically, and socioeconomically diverse samples.

References

Ali, J. I., Smart, C. M., & Gawryluk, J. R. (2018). Subjective cognitive decline and APOE E4: A

systematic review. *Journal of Alzheimer's Disease*, *65*(1), 303–320.

Amariglio, R. E., Townsend, M. K., Grodstein, F., Sperling, R. a, & Rentz, D. M. (2011).

Specific subjective memory complaints in older persons may indicate poor cognitive

function. *Journal of the American Geriatrics Society*, *59*(9), 1612–1617.

https://doi.org/10.1111/j.1532-5415.2011.03543.x

Beard, R. L., & Neary, T. M. (2013). Making sense of nonsense: Experiences of mild cognitive

impairment. *Sociology of Health & Illness*, *35*(1), 130–146.

https://doi.org/10.1111/j.1467-9566.2012.01481.x

Comijs, H. C., Deeg, D. J. H., Dik, M. G., Twisk, J. W. R., & Jonker, C. (2002). Memory

complaints; the association with psycho-affective and health problems and the role of

personality characteristics. A 6-year follow-up study. *Journal of Affective Disorders*, *72*(2),

157–165. https://doi.org/10.1016/S0165-0327(01)00453-0

Derouesné, C., Lacomblez, L., Thibault, S., & LePoncin, M. (1999). Memory complaints in

young and elderly subjects. *International Journal of Geriatric Psychiatry*, *14*(4), 291–301.

https://doi.org/10.1002/(SICI)1099-1166(199904)14:4<291::AID-GPS902>3.0.CO;2-7

Dux, M. C., Woodard, J. L., Calamari, J. E., Messina, M., Arora, S., Chik, H., & Pontarelli, N.

(2008). The moderating role of negative affect on objective verbal memory performance

and subjective memory complaints in healthy older adults. *Journal of the International*

Neuropsychological Society : JINS, *14*(2), 327–336.

https://doi.org/10.1017/S1355617708080363

Edmonds, E. C., Delano-Wood, L., Galasko, D. R., Salmon, D. P., & Bondi, M. W. (2014).

Subjective cognitive complaints contribute to misdiagnosis of mild cognitive impairment. *Journal of the International Neuropsychological Society, 20*(8), 836–847. https://doi.org/10.1017/S135561771400068X

Edmonds, E. C., Delano-Wood, L., Galasko, D. R., Salmon, D. P., & Bondi, M. W. (2015). Subtle cognitive decline and biomarker staging in preclinical Alzheimer's disease. *Journal of Alzheimer's Disease, 47*(1), 231–242. https://doi.org/10.3233/JAD-150128

Elliott, R. (2003). Executive functions and their disorders: Imaging in clinical neuroscience. *British Medical Bulletin, 65*(1), 49–59. https://doi.org/10.1093/bmb/65.1.49

Friedman, C., & Yorio, K. (2006). *The girl's guide to being a boss (without being a bitch): Valuable lessons, smart suggestions, and true stories for succeeding as the chick-in-charge.* New York, NY: Morgan Road Books.

Haavisto, W. (2018). Do individual differences explain discrepancies between subjective memory and objective memory?. *book Abstracts International Section A: Humanities and Social Sciences, 79*(1-A).

Haussmann, R., Sauer, C., Birnbaum, A., & Donix, M. (2019). Gender differences in the perception of cognitive decline. *Asian Journal of Psychiatry, 46,* 6.

Hill, N. L., Mogle, J., Wion, R., Munoz, E., DePasquale, N., Yevchak, A. M., & Parisi, J. M. (2016). Subjective cognitive impairment and affective symptoms: A systematic review. *Gerontologist, 56*(6), e109–e127. https://doi.org/10.1093/geront/gnw091

Jenkins, A., Tree, J. J., Thornton, I. M., & Tales, A. (2019). Subjective cognitive impairment in 55-65-year-old adults is associated with negative affective symptoms, neuroticism, and poor quality of life. *Journal of Alzheimer's Disease, 67*(4), 1367–1378. https://doi.org/10.3233/JAD-180810

Jessen, F., Amariglio, R. E., Buckley, R. F., van der Flier, W. M., Han, Y., Molinuevo, J. L., …
Wagner, M. (2020). The characterisation of subjective cognitive decline. *The Lancet
Neurology, 19*(3), 271–278. https://doi.org/10.1016/S1474-4422(19)30368-0

Jessen, F., Amariglio, R. E., Van Boxtel, M., Breteler, M., Ceccaldi, M., Chételat, G., …
Wagner, M. (2014). A conceptual framework for research on subjective cognitive decline in
preclinical Alzheimer's disease. *Alzheimer's and Dementia, 10*(6), 844–852.
https://doi.org/10.1016/j.jalz.2014.01.001

Lingler, J. H., Nightingale, M. C., Erlen, J. A., Kane, A. L., Reynolds, C. F., Schulz, R., &
DeKosky, S. T. (2006). Making sense of mild cognitive impairment: A qualitive exploration
of the patient's experience. *Gerontologist, 46*(6), 791–800.
https://doi.org/10.1093/geront/46.6.791

McNab, F., Zeidman, P., Rutledge, R. B., Smittenaar, P., Brown, H. R., Adams, R. A., & Dolan,
R. J. (2015). Age-related changes in working memory and the ability to ignore distraction.
Proceedings of the National Academy of Sciences of the United States of America, 112(20),
6515–6518. https://doi.org/10.1073/pnas.1504162112

Merema, M. R., Speelman, C. P., Foster, J. K., & Kaczmarek, E. A. (2013). Neuroticism (not
depressive symptoms) predicts memory complaints in some community-dwelling older
adults. *American Journal of Geriatric Psychiatry, 21*(8), 729–736.
https://doi.org/10.1016/j.jagp.2013.01.059

Miebach, L., Wolfsgruber, S., Frommann, I., Buckley, R., & Wagner, M. (2018). Different
cognitive complaint profiles in memory clinic and depressive patients. *American Journal of
Geriatric Psychiatry, 26*(4), 463–475. https://doi.org/10.1016/j.jagp.2017.10.018

Mulligan, B.P., Smart, C. M., & Ali, J. I. (2016). Relationship of subjective and objective performance indicators in subjective cognitive decline. *Psychology and Neuroscience, 9*(3), 362–378. https://doi.org/10.1037/pne0000061

Pearman, A., & Storandt, M. (2005). Self-discipline and self-consciousness predict subjective memory in older adults. *Journals of Gerontology: Series B Psychological Sciences and Social Sciences*. https://doi.org/10.1093/geronb/60.3.P153

Rabinovici, G. D., Stephens, M. L., & Possin, K. L. (2015). Executive dysfunction. *Continuum: Lifelong Learning in Neurology, 21*(3), 649–659.

Reisberg, B., & Gauthier, S. (2008). Current evidence for subjective cognitive impairment (SCI) as the pre-mild cognitive impairment (MCI) stage of subsequently manifest Alzheimer's disease. *International Psychogeriatrics, 20*(1), 1–16. https://doi.org/10.1017/S1041610207006412

Richard, E., Reitz, C., Honig, L. H., Schupf, N., Tang, M. X., Manly, J. J., … Luchsinger, J. A. (2013). Late-life depression, mild cognitive impairment, and dementia. *JAMA Neurology, 70*(3), 383–389. https://doi.org/10.1001/jamaneurol.2013.603

Shaw, S., & Hoeber, L. (2003). "A strong man is direct and a direct woman is a bitch": Gendered discourses and their influence on employment roles in sports organizations. *Journal of Sport Management, 17*(4), 347–376.

Slavin, M. J., Brodaty, H., Kochan, N. A., Crawford, J. D., Trollor, J. N., Draper, B., & Sachdev, P. S. (2010). Prevalence and predictors of "subjective cognitive complaints" in the Sydney Memory and Ageing Study. *American Journal of Geriatric Psychiatry, 18*(8), 701–710. https://doi.org/10.1097/JGP.0b013e3181df49fb

Smart, C. M., & Krawitz, A. (2015). The impact of subjective cognitive decline on Iowa Gambling Task performance. *Neuropsychology, 29*(6), 971–987.

Snitz, B. E., Lopez, O. L., McDade, E., Becker, J. T., Cohen, A. D., Price, J. C., … Klunk, W. E. (2015). Amyloid-β imaging in older adults presenting to a memory clinic with subjective cognitive decline: A pilot study. *Journal of Alzheimer's Disease*, *48*(S1), S151–S159. https://doi.org/10.3233/JAD-150113

Sperling, R. A., Aisen, P. S., Beckett, L. A., Bennett, D. A., Craft, S., Fagan, A. M., … Phelps, C. H. (2011). Toward defining the preclinical stages of Alzheimer's disease: Recommendations from the National Institute on Aging-Alzheimer's Association workgroups on diagnostic guidelines for Alzheimer's disease. *Alzheimer's and Dementia*, *7*(3), 280–292. https://doi.org/10.1016/j.jalz.2011.03.003

Tobiansky, R., Livingston, G., & Mann, A. (1995). The Gospel Oak Study stage IV: The clinical relevance of subjective memory impairment in older people. *Psychological Medicine, 25*(4), 779–786. https://doi.org/10.1017/S0033291700035029

Tuokko, H. A., & Smart, C. M. (2018). *Neuropsychology of cognitive decline: A developmental approach to assessment and intervention.* New York, NY: Guilford Press.

Vogel, A., Salem, L. C., Andersen, B. B., & Waldemar, G. (2016). Differences in quantitative methods for measuring subjective cognitive decline - Results from a prospective memory clinic study. *International Psychogeriatrics, 28*(9), 1513–1520. https://doi.org/10.1017/S1041610216000272

Wiegand, M. A., Troyer, A. K., Gojmerac, C., & Murphy, K. J. (2013). Facilitating change in health-related behaviors and intentions: A randomized controlled trial of a multidimensional memory program for older adults. *Aging and Mental Health, 17*(7), 808–815. https://doi.org/10.1080/13607863.2013.789000

www.ingramcontent.com/pod-product-compliance
Lightning Source LLC
LaVergne TN
LVHW042355190726
843493LV00005B/1033